Birth...

journeys in the worlds of motherhood

dr veronica moule

DEMETER

Birth...
journey to the wild depths of motherhood
dr veronica moule
Copyright © 2021 Demeter Press

Demeter Press
2546 10th Line
Bradford, Ontario
Canada, L3Z 3L3
Tel: 289-383-0134
Email: info@demeterpress.org
Website: www.demeterpress.org

Demeter Press logo based on the sculpture "Demeter" by Maria-Luise Bodirsky www.keramik-atelier.bodirsky.de

Printed and Bound in Canada

Cover artwork: Veronica Moule
Typesetting: Michelle Pirovich

Library and Archives Canada Cataloguing in Publication
Title: Birth : ...journey to the wild depths of motherhood / by Veronica Moule.
Other titles: Journey to the wild depths of motherhood
Names: Moule, Veronica, 1968- author.
Identifiers: Canadiana 20200374907 | ISBN 9781772583274 (softcover)
Subjects: LCGFT: Poetry.
Classification: LCC PR9619.4.M68 B57 2021 | DDC 821/.92—dc23

I acknowledge the Dja Dja Wurrung as traditional custodians of the land this was written on, and pay my respects to the Elders past, present and emerging

I acknowledge the First Nations people's connection to country, and that sovereignty was never ceded

I give thanks to Dja Dja Wurrung country, where my sons Aidan, Callum and Ben were born

I give thanks to Wathaurong country, where my son Jarah was born

In this collection, I reference the 'message tree' and 'birthing tree'. I write from my experience sitting in stillness with these trees, as a non-indigenous woman.

I honour the stories of birth and community held in country, in culture.

'be gentle on this land
a child was born here'

Archie Roach
Gunditjmara / Bundjalung

4 times I have birthed
reached into the depths of myself
my wonder
my self-observation
my raw
wild
passionate
determined
she-wolf

contents

together we climb the mountain
because I climb this mountain for you
together we wade through the river
together we shelter in the trees
gathered with my support crew
or standing solo
exuding the theatrics of the stage
or in the quiet Zen of retreat
I unravel myself
open myself
surrender myself
to this bold and broad and astonishing experience
that will release you
my child
into the world
and will forge my will
my heart
my being
into the wild depths
of motherhood

... I will accept all this child brings
my body
my heart
my mind will stretch
beyond its known boundaries
and I will learn of openness and love
again, and again
unconditional holding of this child
this child who resonates
within the depths of my being...

introduction

N ine months have passed, your beautiful belly has bloomed beyond your imagination. Ten moon cycles your baby has grown, and now, full like the moon, it is time.

Your baby will transition, from being held in your womb to being held in your arms. How will this happen? Do you yearn for natural childbirth?

… Labour … You will stretch beyond your knowing and meet all of yourself. Are you willing to meet all of yourself? The bold warrior, stepping into the rhythm of the beginning of labour – courage to commence. Then the warrior must step aside, over the hours or days it takes to move through the first stages of labour. Step aside to surrender to the awesomeness of the female body. Traversing chaos, enmeshed in pain, stretching beyond logical limits, as the hormones of love and acceptance pulse through your body.

Yet you don't have to. You can by-pass the pain, the stretching, the opening, the hormonal breadths and depths. This has all become unnecessary discomfort with our technological and medical advances. Why would woman want to stretch herself? Why would she want to experience the raw honesty of her body, in an expression like no other? Is there any point in discomfort? Is there any point to this challenge?

Birth was considered a 'rite of passage', this extraordinary shift from woman to mother. Yet we've lost the art of the 'rite of passage'.

It is glorious watching a child learn, the first smile, the first steps. We delight in these turning points in life. Yet once they grow, show signs of maturing into their adult bodies, as the mystery gets bigger, culturally we pull away, embarrassed by the changes.

We don't welcome menarche with ceremony. We rarely acknowledge the day to day impacts of our menstrual cycles. Instead women hide them away as if they don't exist, or modify themselves with hormones, controlling the primitive parts of ourselves.

And that's OK, if that's what a woman wants, but you can't get through natural labour being in control. Control will take you to the warrior, through the beginning stages, but not to the surrender.

Surrender ... we give up, let ourselves be controlled by the more powerful being. It's generally thought of as failure, subjugation to other, loss of autonomy. Yet in labour, it's in surrendering to the power within ourselves that we meet our potency, our strength, our awesome capabilities. The birth of a child can't be completed until we surrender ourselves entirely to the process.

Yet in our hospital structures, what does surrender look like? How does a woman surrender into the potency of her biology, when the system is asking her to surrender to its rules and regulations?

Surveillance, urgency, emergency, scrutiny. This is the system – looking for what could be wrong, creating stress in the process. Worrying about worrying, in the search for the less likely. And it's not just one test, one test leads to more tests that lead to more tests. The consumer knows that ultrasounds are sometimes wrong when guessing the sex of the baby, but that is not the only error. All those numbers, when the 3-D structure of the baby is put on a 2-D screen and measured, have an error rating of 15%. But it's hard to remember that the numbers are inaccurate – they look so neat and precise, so the error rating is forgotten, and the test is repeated over and over. And from this place of inaccuracy, decisions are made by the clinicians about what will happen to women's bodies, if they are 'allowed' to continue the pregnancy, or what interventions 'need' to occur.

What does it mean hormonally, biochemically, to the pregnant body of woman, to be sitting in heightened awareness and fear? They're rarely the woman's fears, but fears that sit in the structure of the hospital system. This is a system that fears missing anything or making a mistake, so searches every corner and crevice of woman, trying to make science answer all the questions of the mystery of a growing child.

How can women feel enhanced by their capability and normality within this surveillance?

And what is normal these days?

Women come from their mothers' groups, and reflect on the plethora of emergency caesareans that follow from inductions of labour. They feel these are the most frequently told birthing stories. Intervention in birth has become the norm. It is normal, in the sense that caesarean section is so common that it has become a standard mode of birth; but there is nothing normal, in a biological sense, to women having their pregnancies induced and the baby being surgically removed.

Women who have a natural birth story often feel unable to share their stories in these mothers' groups, silenced in their compassion for women with traumatic birth experiences. And there are women between these two groups – those who had an 'alright' birth, they hear the stories of trauma and think 'my story isn't that bad', so they package away their 'OK birth' into a place of acceptance, until the next pregnancy invites them to confront the idea of labour and birth again.

How did we get to this place in birthing culture? In the healthcare system, we like to think we're working in 'evidence-based medicine', and sometimes we are – particularly when the evidence supports further investigation and intervention. We analyse in peer-reviewed meetings, try and foresee how we could have managed someone a bit better, and be more prepared next time.

Yet, not everything fits within an evidence-based process. CTGs (monitoring of the baby's heart rate) increase intervention rates in low risk women, without improvements in outcomes. This has been known for over 20 years, yet they continue to have a dominant role in birthing services. This isn't an evidence based response, it is a cultural and institutional response. Whilst birthing services sit within the hospital framework, hospitals will act like hospitals do – monitoring and intervening. This hospital model has been highly successful when managing medical problems.

The difference though, a difference that isn't clear in the language or actions of the hospital, is that childbirth is a normal, physiological experience. It is not, by its very nature, a disease. But it is managed in a structure that is disease focussed, and so is viewed as a disease because that is how the institution works.

And yes, this is now 'normal' because 99% of Australian women give birth in a hospital.

For the last 20 years, I have worked in birthing in a small country town hospital, where the birthing rooms overlook the botanical gardens, and the maternity ward is adjacent to but separated from the acute medical section.

Labour is a wild ride and the soundtrack to this, the song of the labouring woman, sometimes floats down the corridors. Often, we have elderly women in the rooms nearby. To the sound of women in active labour, these elderly women reflect on their own birth experiences. The birth of their children, those moments in life that are not reproducible, the raw power, the wonder as a child entered their lives.

These memories rise, they are accessed easily, because these moments in life are important. These incredible turning points, where some of our greatest challenges are met, and life changes – never to be the same again.

Our culture doesn't value these moments, or honour the importance of them to the woman or the mother-baby dyad. Superficially, we as a culture think it's nice and beautiful, miraculous, when a baby is born; but truly respecting the natural birthing journey of woman, to open from the depths of her being, however she as an individual can do this, is not the agenda of the vast majority of hospital births. For each woman, labour and birth are some of the most important days in her life, and whether she feels honoured or disrespected, she will carry these experiences with her forever.

Statistics show a picture of birth as an accomplishment in medicine and intervention: rising caesarean rates, epidural use, inductions of labour.

Hiding in those statistics, is the fact that one-on-one care with a midwife reduces complications. Continuity of care – receiving care from a known midwife through the pregnancy, labour and birth reduces intervention rates. This has been known for decades, yet our health care system doesn't search for ways to implement this as the foundation of care. The current, mechanised hospital maternity system persists with a model of fractured care that is not woman-centred.

Instead, escalating intervention rates, complications, and costs are being accrued in maternity care. Birthing centres have been absorbed into general labour wards, and the continuity of care model, known to be the most cost-effective and personally fulfilling for women and midwifery staff, has been eroded or ignored.

Why do we do this? Why are hospitals structured like this?

Why is the obstetric model of care so dominant?

Why do we accept a caesarean section rate climbing from 23% in 2000 to 37% in 2019 without active and deep conversations in community forums, feminist groups, the welfare sector, mental health forums, and mothers' groups?

If a woman is looking to birth with intervention, she can find this anywhere. But what can a woman who wants a natural birth, free from intervention, find to support her? Physiological birth of both her baby and placenta. How can the system support women in having a natural birth, and create a space that maximises the efficiency of her physiology? Hospitals work against physiology – cool, clinical, bright lights, mechanised noises, strangers at a time of vulnerability and intimacy.

Why can't hospitals offer women a place of emotional safety, supportive touch with a known midwife, gentle tenderness, a dark, warm place, offerings that enhance her oxytocin? Why can't this be offered through both the labour and birth, and in the time of the first meeting of mother and child?

Physiological third stage is the natural birth of the placenta. Allowing each woman the opportunity to be totally present with her baby, from the moment it is born. Present in body, in mind and in her physiology – to the hormonal symphony that is singing in her system as she births her baby, and for the first hour or so of her baby's life.

A natural, physiological birth can most commonly and safely be followed by a natural, physiological birth of her placenta. This is how birth has worked from the dawn of time and humanity, until about 50 years ago, when hospitals started using synthetic oxytocin (Syntocinon) for the delivery of the placenta.

I once worked with a midwife who told me the story: 'I'm so old, I remember the time before Syntocinon. We used to wait for an hour for the placenta. Then Syntocinon came along, and we'd give the injection, and the placenta would come out, it was great, we could finish tidying everything up.'

This is a story about how Syntocinon made the maternity ward work more efficiently. She didn't talk about radical changes in bleeding rates, she reflected on how it made her job easier. Syntocinon is a vitally useful medication in the treatment of excess blood loss. Routine use, where every woman receives this medication after her child is born, was embraced because it made the hospital work more efficiently. And now, 50 years down the track, all midwives and doctors working in maternity have been trained in the system of routine use of synthetic oxytocin for delivery of the placenta. It sits in their place of clinical norm, of comfort, and if challenged by a woman requesting a natural placental birth, most midwives and doctors feel fear – they haven't been taught how to 'manage' this. And from this place of fear, they layer their concerns on the possibility of bleeding, bleeding that can be managed with medical treatments. Studies show that when women are supported to have truly physiological placental births, they do not have greater rates of bleeding.

What is the urgency, that health care workers 'need' to come between a mother and her child from the first moment it is born? Hormonally separate the two. Why do we think this is culturally acceptable?

If we were to watch an animal documentary, or if we viewed our pets deliver their babies, and another of that species came and pushed between the mother and baby, we would be shocked, horrified. We would wonder if the mother would be able to attach properly with the baby, if she would imprint her child to ensure its survival.

Supporting a woman having a physiological third stage is not difficult. All it takes is quietness and respect. It offers an opportunity to birth workers to pause and breathe into the wonder of birth – to feel the love in the room, to feel honoured to have been part of such a special and intimate moment. I usually sit quietly, write some notes, keep an eye on her blood loss, enjoy the joy in the room.

And whilst the roar of labour has subsided, the hormonal response in the mother hasn't. She is experiencing the biggest peak of oxytocin in her whole life. More than the surges of oxytocin that caused the waves of contractions that took her through labour and birth, more than the oxytocin peaks when she has intimate orgasmic moments with her partner. This is meant to be the greatest oxytocin moment in her life, but we interfere and dampen this moment with a dose of synthetic oxytocin.

What is the purpose of oxytocin, this exquisite hormone, that opens ourselves to falling deeply, madly, orgasmically in love? The challenge and pain of labour is astonishing, and not many women associate birth with orgasm. Yet this is the hormonal basis of birth, oxytocin is the hormone of love, the hormone of uterine contractions, the hormone that imprints our baby into our brains, the hormone of ecstasy and orgasm.

Is this the problem? Do we, as a society, still think that women don't or shouldn't orgasm? How confronting is it to suggest that the hour after birth could be more ecstatic for nearly every woman than it currently is?

Giving synthetic oxytocin could be considered an outrageous intrusion on a women's hormonal life, at the biggest and most intense time in her life.

Only 1.5% of Australian women have a physiological birth of her placenta.

A pregnant woman came to see me, returning to her home town to have her baby. She was 30 weeks pregnant at our first antenatal consultation, and as I checked the size of her belly and the direction the baby was lying in, she said 'that's the first time someone has touched my tummy, the OBG in New York just used the ultrasound every time.'

Touch. Our first moments, our first sense. In utero, we are enveloped by the touch of the womb. The tiny flutters, like butterfly wings, mother's first sense of her baby moving, that strengthen with time. As baby kicks inside, mother feels for her baby, her hands pretending to reach through her body layers, sending back to baby her conscious touch.

Why is our society so out of touch about birth? Losing connection with natural birth, disconnected from others, from self, in this complex world of technology. The touch received in hospitals, the touch midwives and doctors are trained to give, is clinical touch – checking the pulse, the blood pressure cuff, assessment of the strength of contractions, vaginal examinations, IV catheter needles. And with any luck, some hand holding.

But there's more to touch, touch that can show humanity as well as clinical skills. Gentle sharing, strength in togetherness, feel support, lean into it, let yourself go, feel safe, relax into caring touch, loving touch, gentle intimacy. In labour, touch can help facilitate the woman's opening, expansion, release. Gentle, present touch, helps us relax into our bodies, slows the chatter of the mind. This is how we relax, how we allow, how we find a way to loosen our fears, to open ourselves. In natural childbirth, women must open themselves to allow the passage of the baby out.

But we're 'out of touch' in our busyness. Australian hospital structures demand pen on paper. The culture and rhythm and ritual circuiting the pregnant woman is not from the feminine, it's not the rhythm of woman, it is around the hospital's needs. And women file through the staccato of hospital rhythm, and try their best to fit in, modify themselves...out of touch with themselves and their needs.

When 7 months pregnant with my 4th child, I was invited to speak at a conference. I prepared a talk about the emotional preparation of woman prior to birthing her baby, using the ancient story of Persephone, from Greek mythology, as an illustration of the process of pre-labour, labour and birth.

The story of Persephone's journey into the underworld is emblematic of the steps women must undertake to birth within our patriarchal cultural structure.

This story is from the times of early agriculture, a representation of the cycles of the solar calendar, of the seasons, of sowing and growing and harvesting the grain until a time of fallow. This time in humanity's history, the development of agriculture, is also the turning point in power relations from matriarchal or egalitarian to patriarchal societies. The shift from hunter gatherers, where the women gathered and the men hunted; to domestication of animals and development of agricultural skills in planting and managing the soil, invited a new way of being. Women continued to plant and gather, to cook and provide the basis of the care of the community. Men, liberated from time spent hunting, continued to manage animals – through fencing and 'animal husbandry'. Through fencing, men defined ownership of land, with resultant control of women. Men, freer with their time, utilised this in developing politics – the structures and definitions that the community were to now live by.

The story of Persephone comes from this time, this turning point in community structures. It is a story of fertility in the harsh and controlling structures of patriarchy (Zeus and Hades), the grief of loss (Demeter), the vulnerability of the maiden (Kore) as she navigates both light and dark, and her success in straddling both worlds as woman (Persephone), albeit tethered to the patriarchal structures.

This is the reality of our cultural construct. That for women to stretch themselves through both light and dark, to succeed in the birth of themselves as women and mothers, women now do this within a patriarchal structure. With all the respect and disrespect that it can muster, for a man will never understand the complexities of being woman. In many ways, women also don't understand this – as part of 'the dark' is an embodied sense of self that is non-literal, not logical, beyond cognition. Women can move through their pre-menstrual times every month, in a state of confusion or irritation, yet not be able to identify the coming bleed until it arrives – month after month, year after year, decade after decade. How exquisitely non-rational.

Labour is non-literal, it's not logical. It is from this non-rational part of ourselves that we give birth. The cognitive mind is the least useful organ for labour – it brings us awareness, alertness, into our fright-flight. Women labour better in the dark, because labour is of this 'dark' part, the unknown or unknowable part of woman.

Birth workers observe women, we listen to the sounds of labouring women. We can also feel changes in our bodies, changes that mirror the labouring woman's body. I work in an embodied way, I breathe into the depths of myself, as a midwife. I can feel the contractions, feel the opening, feel the call to wait – as it is not yet time, my body helps me know where this individual woman is in her labour. It is a form of meditation that all birth workers can nurture. It is a meditation that invites us to listen to the 'dark' parts of ourselves, our non-cognitive selves, and be guided through her labour by our inner knowing.

The following collection of poems was initiated by my fight to maintain physiological third stage. This has been part of my practice for over 20 years. I was asked by the hospital to stop because it was 'not being done elsewhere.' Yet in this world of evidence based medicine, the hospital administration didn't want to know my evidence. They didn't want to know the statistics that support this as a safe and appropriate practice. Hospitals listen to evidence that supports their culture of practice, that fits within their structure, where they can define what women are 'allowed' to do – from a position of patronising control, not respectful consent.

This was a fight, a fight for women's rights to have their voices heard, to be respected in their choices in childbirth. It was a fight for the right to not assault women, by administering a medication she did not want, that she did not consent to. Women are assaulted in the name of medicine every day in our birthing services. They are bullied and coerced, until they agree to the hospital's way of treating them, 'managing them'. Women are emotionally manipulated by hospitals, they are told they will die, or their baby will die if they don't follow the recommended treatment. Yet this very rarely happens, and there are many steps hospitals can take to ensure the physical safety of women and babies, whilst also listening to and supporting women in their requests.

This collection of poems arose from birthing experiences, and from my advocacy of women's choices – reasonable yet maybe unusual choices from the institution's perspective. Through this fight, I travelled to the depths of myself, to the breadth of myself, gave air to the uncompromising fire in me, that melted away my insulation, until I found the breath in me, over and over again. Some poems are autobiographical. Some were written in anger and disgust at the system, some written on my hands and knees rocking back and forth like a labouring woman, they are messages from the depths of my being, offering clarity.

We start where all women now begin their birth journey – with Zeus, in the structure of patriarchy. Then we move beyond, through the supportive hold of mother Demeter, then further into ourselves until we find the unique wonder of woman, and the breath and calm and ecstasy that she can hold.

The Story of Persephone

Zeus, the father of the gods, has a sister, Demeter, goddess of mother earth and a brother Hades, god of the underworld. Demeter and Zeus have a daughter, the maiden Kore. Hades fell in love with Kore and asked Zeus if he could marry her.

Zeus feared offending his brother Hades. Zeus also knew Demeter would never forgive him if Hades married Kore, and committed Kore to the underworld. Zeus neither agreed or refused, so Hades planned to abduct her.

Kore was gathering flowers one day, when the earth suddenly opened and Hades appeared, in a chariot drawn by 4 black horses. He grabbed Kore, and returned through the chasm in the earth.

Demeter came to collect her daughter, but couldn't find her anywhere. Distraught and desperate, she searched high and low, and travelled to the furthest corners of the earth.

A messenger told Demeter to approached Helios, the sun god who sees everything.

Helios said it was Hades, with the connivance of Zeus. Demeter was so angry, that instead of returning to Olympus, she wandered the earth, forbidding the trees to fruit or herbs to grow.

Famine was so great, that humans were in danger of extinction.

Zeus feared there would be nobody left to make offerings to the gods, and begged for reconciliation.

Demeter refused, she swore the earth be barren until Kore was returned.

Zeus sent a message to Hades requesting Kore's return.

Kore had refused to eat or drink since her abduction.

Hades said to Kore that she could return home.

Kore's tears ceased, but as she was leaving she ate 7 seeds from the pomegranate.

Kore returned to the light and was joyfully embraced by Demeter, but when Demeter heard she had eaten the pomegranate she grew dejected and sad. Kore had eaten the fruit of the underworld, and must stay in the underworld forever.

Rhea, mother of Zeus, Demeter and Hades, proposed a compromise that would restore fertility to the land.

It was decided that Kore would spend 3 months of each year in Hades' company as Persephone, queen of the underworld, and the remaining 9 months with Demeter.

dr veronica moule

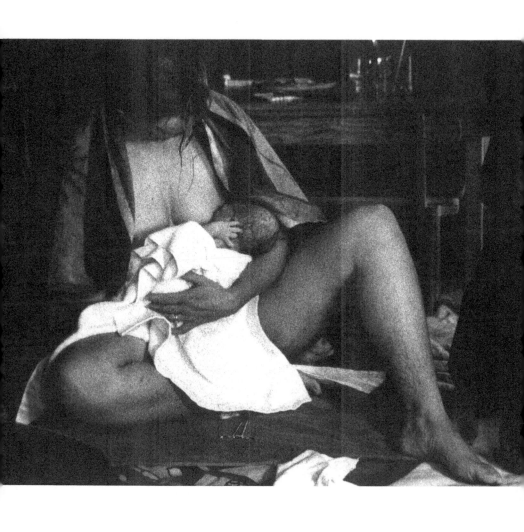

unfolding

labour

how do we unfold
unravel ourselves
this outrageously awesome journey
of our bodies opening
when a child is born

we are the responsible parents
with strength in self
secure footings
despite the medical system's patronising behaviour
we must stand in our strength

Demeter calls
we search for our mothers
our sisters
mother earth
to hold us as we open
yet we alone will birth our child

and who are we?
which parts need unravelling
who is the raw, pure woman
who holds presence with herself
knows and trusts herself
to mother this child
together, mother and child searching for their dance and song

she knows this child will come
that the journey of labour will be hard
maybe the hardest days of her life

so she drops into herself
warrior woman
courage to commit to the process
this labour and birth
labour of love

and the prize is big
almost too much
a child will come
it's too much to lose
vulnerability rises
there is no escape

you'll be tested to the depths of your heart
the depths of your soul
and find the depths of your capacity
devotion
the full and aching heart

we must trust
the burning fire of birth
surrender
to this centuries-old rite of passage…

until we are open
open to the overwhelming love
of a mother for her child
pulsing with love hormones
imprinting love
boundless togetherness
searching in wonder
for this miraculous unfolding
birth

Persephone,
story of woman

the unravelling and reforming of woman
let go of father's hold
beyond mother's embrace
searching for self
in darkness and light
from girl to woman
from pregnant woman to mother
Persephone
the story of woman

Zeus

---

paternal

safety

security

structure

restraint

limitations

caution

patriarchy

responsibility

safety, security

we are the responsible parents
with strength in self
despite the medical system's patronising behaviour
we must stand in our strength

how are we physically held?
what is our structure
we step into the monolith
concrete structures, concrete views
surveillance through ultrasounds
is your body performing adequately?
is your body about to fail?
do we need to step in?
rescue your baby from the limitations of your body
this is the current world of childbirth
induction of labour, epidurals, caesarians
the rules held tight
despite women's individual desires

what is the physical structure of each woman's body
her pelvis, her soft tissues, her fascia
how does her body hold her baby
is baby free to be in optimal position
or is her body pulling tight
making her baby lie posterior, asynclitic
how does a baby navigate
through a tight and frozen pelvis
confusion reigns
things are not smooth
rhythm is lost
...the system can rescue

do you feel safe?
do you need every piece of equipment that is ever used available?
can you trust their decision making?
does it feel wise?

dr veronica moule

disease

having a baby is not easy
there's nothing easy about it
but it's not dis-ease either
natural birthing isn't about ease-disease

hospitals

women search for normal birth
for this incredible experience
where they conquer the mountain of labour
the biggest test of their life
and welcome a baby into their family

hospitals hold tight rules and structures
they are a culture within themselves
that doctors and midwives work within
aiming to bring the best outcomes

and what is the best outcome?
from the hospital's perspective, it is a live mother and baby
preferably with a low morbidity
and hospitals can look at the minutiae of clinical indices
and try to achieve these outcomes
we look through CTGs and ultrasounds and other interventions
interventions with wide discrepancies in their accuracy and
    predictability
because these are the tools that we have
and the more tools we collect,
the more we seem to think the tools hold the key

and what is the best outcome for women and families?
to be able to walk into birth feeling supported
supported to the depth that she feels that
she has the capability to open her body
and birth her baby
feeling supported to make informed decisions about her care,
rather than being given information and assuming consent

dr veronica moule

best outcome is when a woman gives birth
and the family embraces their child
and they step back into the world
enriched by this experience
ready to traverse the complexity of mothering and parenting

and evidence exists to support women and the hospitals in their
    desires
one-on-one care with a known midwife reduces morbidity
and supports women in strengthening their sense of capacity
we've known this for years
midwives bring support and better outcomes
CTGs and ultrasounds bring interventions
and intervention rates have soared
but mortality rates are much the same
and morbidity rates are increasing
and we know the answer
why can't we listen to the answer?
what is the point of evidence
if we take no notice of it

if we were to have an evidence-based support structure
then midwives would be respected
as the experts of normal
and they would teach women about normal birth
and they would teach doctors about normal birth
and hospitals would create structures that support midwives in
    providing one-on-one care
and roster them well
and care for them
and hospitals and AHPRA would respect independent midwives
who are experts in normal
and when they recognise abnormal, and more care is required
welcome them into their structures
because we all want to provide the best care

average, usual, normal and natural in birth,
shouldn't they all be the same thing
shouldn't an average woman expect a completely normal natural
    birth
wouldn't evolution bring us to that expectation
but no, natural birth is no longer the normal, usual or average
    experience
and women don't know this
women go to their health service in good faith
expecting direction and advice to help them have a natural birth
but no, the health service with a full range of policies and
    procedures
direct women to an average birth, the new normal,
with every intervention available
and intervention almost always used.

the caesarean section rate is rising
and in some hospitals, it's more than 50% of births
and women aren't told these statistics
how can they make an informed decision about their place of birth
how can women place themselves in the institution,
where what they want is a normal or usual outcome
if they don't know these statistics?
how can we support hospitals with good statistics?
what and how can we learn from practitioners with good statistics?

in the striving for improving outcomes,
the outcomes are worsening
and in part this may be demographic change
as older and more obese women are birthing
but statistically this doesn't explain all of the change
the more institutions rely on ineffective or inaccurate tools,
the further we seem to get from lessening morbidity
and the harder it is for new midwifery and medical graduates
to understand truly normal birth

dr veronica moule

the postpartum haemorrhage rate was 10-15% 20yrs ago, now it
    sits at 25%
the induction of labour rate was 20% 25yrs ago, now it's 28%

we have random targets (eg determining baby growth)
changing goalposts (eg blood sugar levels)
more intervention
worse morbidity
no changes to mortality

we're not heading in the right direction
the more obstetric we get,
the more obstetrics is required
somehow, we need to turn around
we need to become more midwifery
then more midwifery will be required
and morbidity levels will drop
and families will be able to embrace their child and their future
as more confident, capable and functional parents

risk aversion

there is a continual shift in birthing services to increasing
    intervention
this is what the statistics say
this is what women say, who come to debrief their birth
    experience
we are losing any sense of risk tolerance
the more risk averse we become
the less patient autonomy
for some women this is fine –
there are women who want to absent themselves from labour
they call for an epidural early
and they are well catered for in the public and the private sector
Victoria's current epidural rate is 40%

for women who don't want to absent themselves
women who want to be present for this astonishing experience of
    labour
the biggest event of their life
how do we support them?
they don't want to slip into the intervention model for no good
    reason
they do have opinions about their care
they have their own personal philosophies – religious or spiritual
they have their own emotional challenges that make them bold,
    or anxious, or angry, or passive or stubborn
and this can make it difficult as a birth attendant
difficult to reach them for their emotional needs
difficult to understand where they are coming from
truly respecting a woman's choice means that sometimes we as
    birth attendants need to sit in difficult and uncomfortable places

dr veronica moule

there is a vulnerability as birth attendants
we practice simulated scenarios of obstetric emergencies
but we don't really want to do these in real situations
and it's not until we face these clinical situations
that we find out what our capacity is
we hope, but we don't know, if we'll be calm and mature
and follow the protocol from memory
or, we've had these experiences
and we couldn't overcome our fear
somebody else stepped into our place
or the outcome was poor
and we fear this ever happening again
so we tolerate less risk in the next woman

we are searching for risk factors
searching with tools that are not very accurate
then we're believing these inaccurate tools
we are being risk averse
if we're clever we might find something
before it would present itself clinically
and the earlier things are modified
the earlier interventions are put in place
this is happening in pregnancy –
well before labour starts
in fact, the minority of women having a baby start with
    spontaneous labour

there is all this intervention going on
and women have almost no say in whether they participate
because if they don't, they'll be labelled 'difficult patients'
hospitals like obedient patients
hospitals don't like disobedient or difficult patients
'they make you feel naughty if you don't agree with what they're
    recommending'
and hospitals express this,

as though the patient has opened an emotional wound in the
    hospital staff by disagreeing
by women asking for something that is deeply important to them
then these women avoid coming in
they wait until the last minute
and they present us with the florid clinical situations we didn't
    want to deal with
because they feel marginalised
we need to offer health care to these marginalised women
we need to find the way to make them feel some level of safety
and the way intervention rates are going,
marginalised women are not just those the hospital thinks are
    extreme
now any woman wanting to have a truly natural birth,
without unnecessary intervention,
is a marginalised woman

the less we allow women's autonomy
and the more interventions we put in place earlier
as clinicians, our internal goal posts start to modify
our sense of the breadth of normal reduces,
because we don't allow the same breadth within normal
and we are running towards risk aversion...
with minimal tolerance of any risk
and no room for women's decision making,
for women to have a sense of their capability

for women to have allowed themselves to stretch to their own
    breadth of capacity
stretch themselves physically and emotionally
unravel themselves to their depths
to the raw openness physically, emotionally and biochemically
that our biology is designed for
that allows the overwhelming wonder of the mother receiving her
    child for the first time
receiving her child from herself, from within her own body

on a hormonal and cellular level
that primes the mother baby unit
for the rest of their life together
and we can't see what we are losing
as we run towards this risk aversion model of care

op position

birthing an anterior baby feels like climbing a mountain,
with endurance and breath
the path will unfold

birthing a posterior baby is like climbing a mountain
but there is never a path
there are jagged rocks to clamber over
some without footholds
and sometimes I feel like I'm climbing down before going up again
I can't see the summit
I just know there is more mountain

there's an internal chaos with a posterior birth
the pain is big
the sounds are loud
and sometimes they sound like they're leading somewhere
but my inner knowing is confused
that beautiful step by step deepening into myself isn't there
I'm looking sideways for an answer instead of inwards

until the beautiful moment
my baby reaching my pelvic floor and turning
my voice dropping to that deep resonance
ah, now I know this pathway

dr veronica moule

policy

here we go, the start of the year
it's only taken 2 days to show its flavour
and I'm roaring about policy
about the policy we'll need to implement the policy
then that policy will probably need a preliminary policy
'the policies are there to protect the staff'
what are we being protected from? making any decisions?
do we need to run to daddy policy to see if a woman can stand to
    birth?
do we really need to tidy our rooms so much before he gets home;
that there was no evidence of existence, of play, of humanity?
'inside their lonely castles, broken hearts will dwell'
we're working inside the lonely castle of policy
no room for breath
no room for heart
no room for loving

policy, police, same origin
let's turn maternity into a police state
for our own protection
protect us from those normal women
with their benign requests
I want to feed my child breast milk, donated
I want to stay in the bath until crowning
I want to birth my baby in the bath

and if something goes wrong, we'll all run to policy
to protect us from the evil gaze
of the patriarchal medical hierarchy
looking for their pawns to eat

in their weird chess game of box ticking
and the responsibility falls on me
what is it, that makes some midwives trust policy over me?
my stats are good, they are better than policy's stats, state stats
why don't we recognise the capable practitioners
what is the collective anxiety, the fear of the edge
women travel there every time they labour and birth
yet we try and hold them back from their experience, their wishes
because someone with a clipboard somewhere likes a smoother
    edge
can't breathe to any stretch of normal
so sucks the oxygen out of women

theme

there is a theme, and I can see it

the structure isn't a worthy decision maker
my woman needs her voice – to speak, and sing and scream her
way through

I was fortunate with my first birth
I did help define that fortune –
place yourself in a setting where what you want is the normal,
and you're more likely to get what you're searching for

I rallied against the hierarchies with my second pregnancy
and my woman surrendered in strength and succeeded

my body was the structural inhibition with my third labour
and my woman accepted the chaos and succeeded

and I rallied against the institution of homebirth midwife guru for
my fourth labour
my woman sang clearly to me,
and she succeeded

and my woman will sing and speak and scream if required
for other women,
to allow their voice in our structure and institution

patriarchal woman

who are you
older woman
emotionally blunted
acting as authority
jumping to conclusions
never asking for the story, the background
instant authority
patronisingly confident
although you've never had this experience

women in power
upholding foreign rules
not tailored to place
or woman
judgemental of our care
our connection
despite our management being appropriate

patriarchy doesn't let things lie
patronising belief of control over women
no respect for informed consent
no recognition of capacity, capability, my depth of responsibility
my ferocious warrior woman is not resting
you've met her before
she mistressed success
now other voices heed the ferocious warrior woman
she is articulate
her arguments stand strong
yours are based on your fear
your compliance, your complicity

dr veronica moule

rumouring with others who enjoy their power
and maybe fear the ferocious warrior woman
so, build a big stone wall
hoping I'll tire throwing myself at it

pelvic instability

how do women
whose pelvises are in shock
who can't move or flex
can't bend or rotate
to support the birth process
because they will break,
how do they open to the vulnerability of birth?
how can they,
if they dissolve in the process
frozen in their bodies afterwards?

how can they connect with their baby
when they have lost their foundation
lost deep in their bones
lost to feeling present, open or capable

I feel thankful that morphine is there
after-birthing morphine
to take away the pain of the body,
that all-consuming pain that doesn't allow another focus
the pain that calls so loudly
that the mother cannot see her baby
relieve that pain
then woman can connect with her baby

dr veronica moule

man

what is the role
of man at birth
his child coming
from the depths of woman
woman opening herself
in a way no man could imagine with his body

woman looking to woman for guidance
or looking within herself
man as bystander
gentle man
wanting to be helpful
practical support
witness to his partner's awesomeness
more awesome than either can imagine

is this the new rite-of-passage to fatherhood?

how do we hold men
through the birth process
welcome them
include them
allow them to shine their capacity
to be of service
humbled
strengthened by the strength of woman
the wonder of woman
strengthened in their capacity to love

healing

where do we ache
our grief from past
measured for management
of our day to day
and the cycles swing
throwing us to our depths
where our pain and wonder and hope reside
wishing for a different story
not necessarily a happier ending
as the physical completions have been fine
a gentler process
requiring less processing

precision, clarity...wait, it's coming...
space from children...time to go
stillness in meditation...warmth of the car
black cockatoos
waters break...transition from car
walk...wait...eyes closed...music near
navigating corridors...pressure in pelvis
staff fear time and distance
but we know nothing of this
standing in the depths of contractions

standing
standing up for your rights
standing with friends and strangers
woman at the edge of time
the edge of her world

'don't take my baby away'
words from the depths
from the past
though very present
flex and bend institution
find another way to breathe
into respect
how do we find the way to say 'yes'
to woman's wants
woman's needs
keep woman as decision-maker
help her heal the past

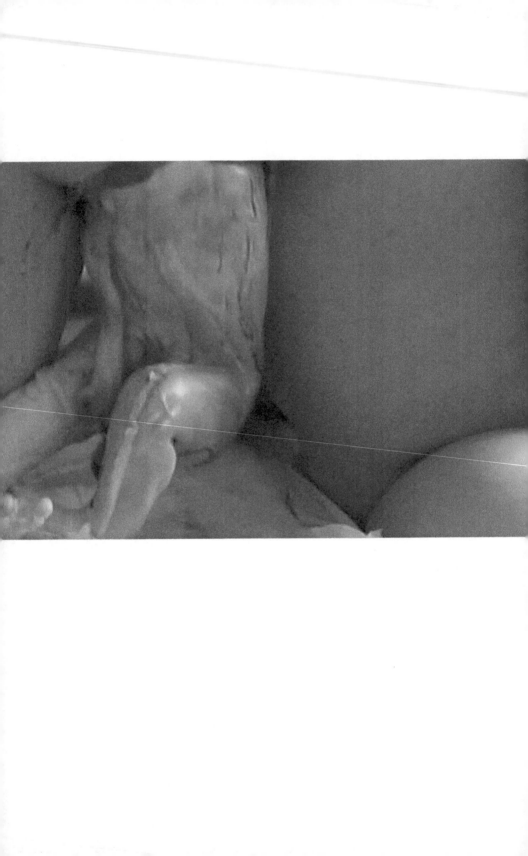

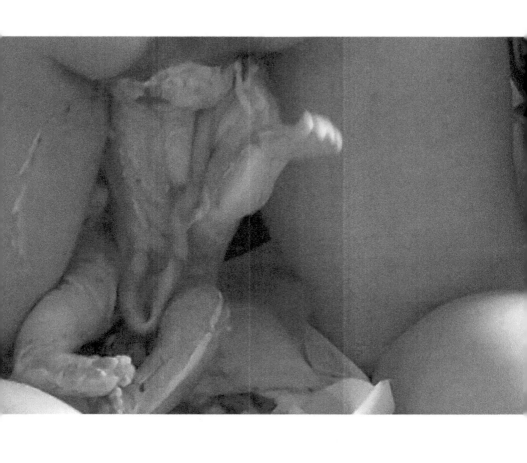

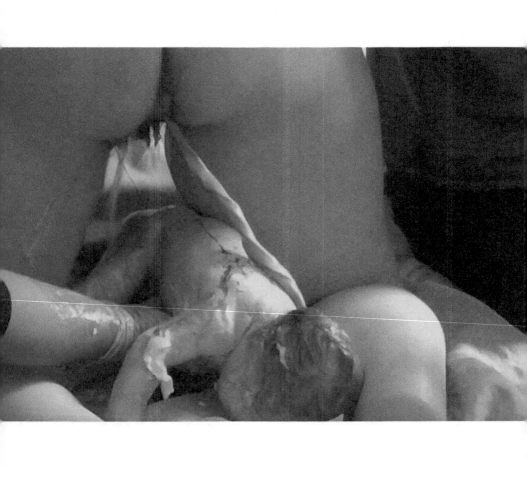

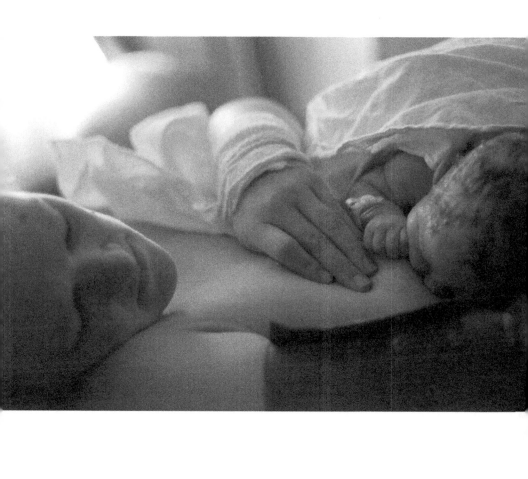

Demeter

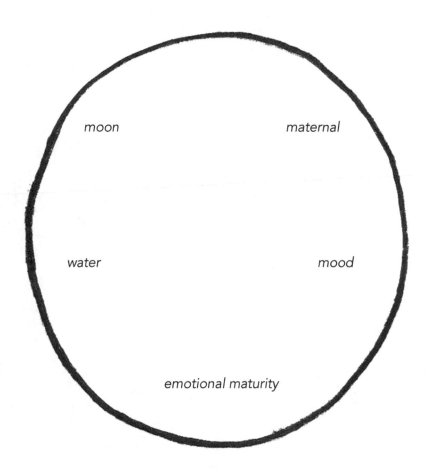

moon   maternal

water   mood

emotional maturity

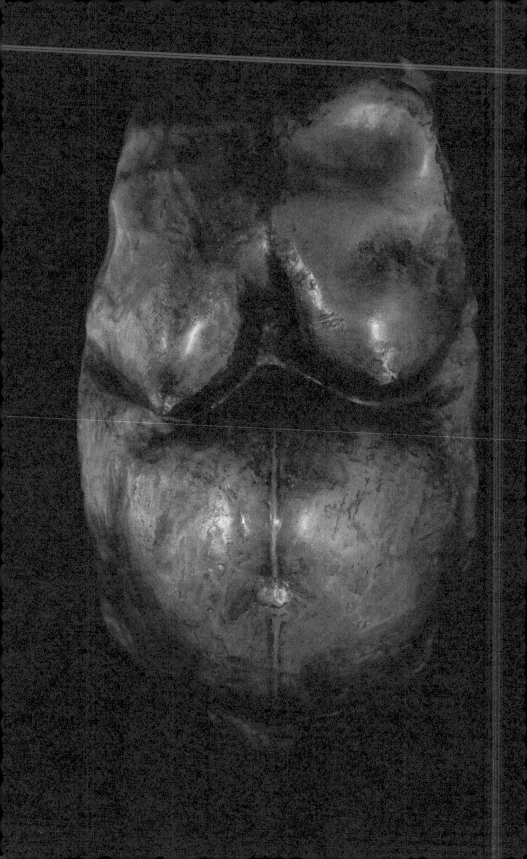

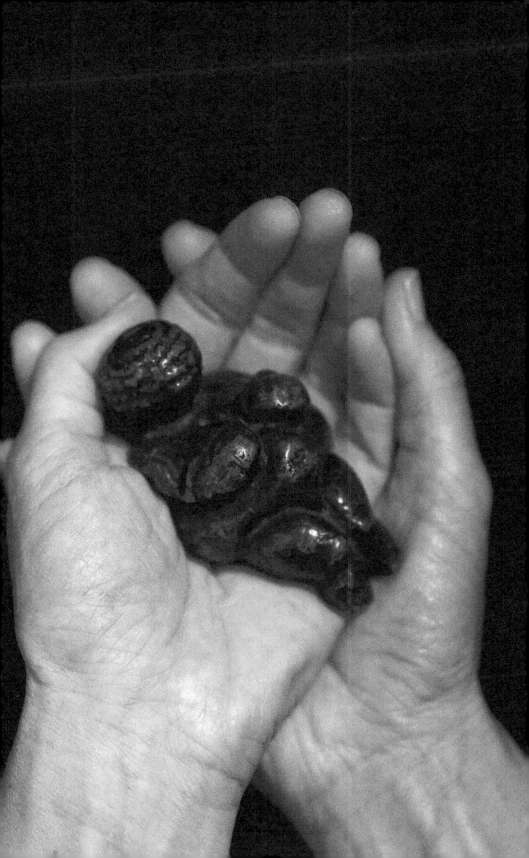

Demeter

hold me in the bosom of woman
wise woman
who has travelled this path to motherhood

grandmother

mother

sister

Mother Mary

Goddess

Isis

Demeter

Kali

Shakti

Papatuanuku

Mother earth

dr veronica moule

moonchild

welcome child
whoever you are
entering this life, this family
and we pour our hopes and aspirations over you
like a cloak
or family arms

this moon brought a child
this super-moon, blue moon, blood moon, lunar eclipse
secluded from sight by the rushing clouds
mystical glimpses of the presence of the hidden light
a child born
through the raw awakening
of a woman held in watery gentleness
togetherness with breath and presence

this moon brought a child
not for the wonder of hope and aspiration
although that will come
but for the wonder of presence
maybe all babies start this way
the wonder of life
capturing these moments
our moments of presence with the profound
before we slip into structures
ways of behaving and being
trying to align directions to our hopes and aspirations
yet wishing for reconnection
with breath
with presence

maternal yearnings

in my preparation for new maternity
emotionally raw,
and soon to be physically raw and open
I yearn for my mother
the one I will soon be
who perceives my emotional, spiritual and physical needs
the one who respects me as a mother now,
and a new mother to be
I yearn for the ideal mother who I am aiming to be
as there is disappointment in the reality
she is afraid to feel, or ask of my needs
welcome babe, into our wider dysfunctional family
I aim to support your emotional needs

dr veronica moule

matrilineal

today I danced with my great grandmother
we danced for her daughter
my grandmother

and we danced for my grandmother's daughter
my mother

and we danced for my mother's daughter
for myself

and we danced for the universal daughters

I haven't birthed daughters
there isn't a singular focus
I danced for all the daughters
for the next generation of women

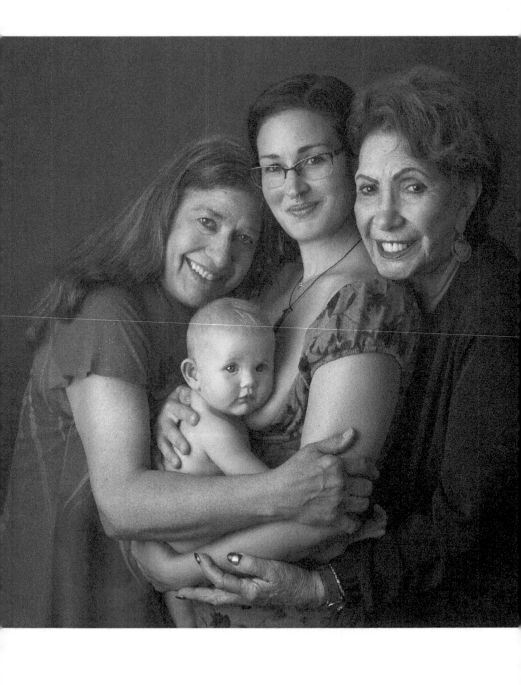

generations

women look back
through their fear
to their mother's birth stories
and if the story was of trauma
of caesarean
there can be a passive resignation
'destined to be repeated'

why don't we look back properly?
not just to recent challenge
look back to the mountain of success
generations of women
60 000 years of natural birth
3 000 generations of vaginal birth

that's legacy
capability
the natural capacity of woman
there's an earth-full of success
women's bodies
through famine and hardship
through abundance
succeeding in labour and birth

water

fire, wild and hot
stand too close
I know I'll be burnt
too far away, and a chill could descend
fluid, where are my watery depths
shallow or deep
it's hard to judge
cascading maybe
step by step
plunging deeper into myself
hoping I'll find clarity
a clear pool for reflection
transparent
somewhere in my depths or shallows

unedited truths
swirling into the waters of self
stirred into my whirlpool's central focus
then sucked back to the depths
of the drainpipe's release
water, water everywhere
dark cloudy skies
wet underfoot
sloshing wetlands
happy ducks
immersion
into my watery realm
boundless, fluid
my calm before my storm?
treading water
waiting for the tide to turn

dr veronica moule

and water puts out fire
and fire turns water to steam
released into the air
I'm kind of hoping to be released into air
to the lightness of breath
blown by the breeze
like a feather or a kite
singing through the leaves of the she-oak
until I find my place on earth again
but first water needs to moisten my soil
that's where the abundance of life is formed

reflection

sometimes we sit in stillness
poised
on the pier
or in the boatshed
levitating
above the watery depths below
maybe holding onto the rational mind
the intellect
not quite prepared to dive
into the depths of emotion
of catharsis

but this scene is not catharsis
it is stillness
gentleness
reflection
we often can't reflect
on stormy waters
in wild seas
that's where we ride the waves
of our wounded selves
gasping for breath
for capacity
to feel grounded
on those heaving boardwalks
awash with salty water,
tears of mother earth

dr veronica moule

gentle reflection
the gift of acceptance
the pause
the moments of stillness
before the wind picks up
and the image is lost
in the chaos of life

catharsis

catharsis
searching our depths
open, exposed
vulnerable

and then review
patterns of behaviour
patterns of communication
and miscommunication   .
judgements
assumptions
and time passes
and we change
but the patterns are strong
we're stretching them to their limits
these old patterns don't suit the change
the catharsis
coping strategies formed in vulnerability
and the vulnerability changes
they demand different answers
different responses

dr veronica moule

now we're unravelling our strategies
claiming personality traits
trying to shift and rumble our habits
habits – set in monthly cycles
and the full moon beams down on us
with her broad moody smile
and enlightens our night-time
with grey light
there's nothing black and white happening
just a swirling greyness

Messenger

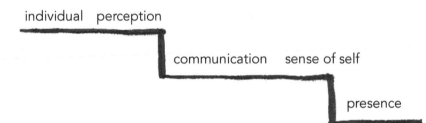

individual   perception

communication   sense of self

presence

messenger

who am I
beyond mother and partner
beyond sister and daughter
who is the pure me
the true individual
can I trace back to my raw self
separate from my other parts
find the place of clarity
of creativity
the place of breath
where I will birth from

I can't labour as partner
I can't birth whilst mothering
I'll labour and birth as the pure woman that I am
beyond family
beyond construct
beyond culture
from the depths of myself as woman

girls

we hold little girls tight
protect them
with kindness
and don't know how to release them
allow them to mature to women
we hold them tighter
as tight as a baby

come
invite my little girl to play
she taught herself
to walk and run
to sing and cry
and roar
before structures moulded her
into something good
and manageable

why would woman choose
to lie on her back to birth
like a submissive puppy
or a baby who can't roll over
look I'm cute, come tickle me
even a 2 year old
will roll away when challenged
onto their hands and knees
like a wild animal
position of catharsis
of release
ready

dr veronica moule

woman unfolds in labour
back to her unmanageable self
she found herself when she learnt to walk and run
and cry and roar
and she'll find herself giving birth
unmoulded

woman

this is the woman that I am
I'm not much interested in living in the box
even though my work and life structure is from there
women, together we can find a way to climb out
and dance freely
in honour of ourselves
our inner women
the bits that laugh deeply
and sing clearly
and allow the birth song to rise and fall
and carry us through
with intensity and trust
to the completions that bring about
our birthing
our rebirthing

message tree

what secrets do you hold
with your crossing limbs
cuddled up
like conjoined twins
growing together
limbs of different orientation
directed pathways
and growth continues
enmeshed together
bridges of branches
storytelling secrets
I wonder how we listen
to your words

unknown destinations

maybe, it's not clear
the purpose
the goal
what I think is the answer
the finish
the end of the cycle
waiting for the reprieve
that doesn't come

I remember holding my son during deep illness
moment to moment,
for many, many months
and when wellness was suggested in his body
and I thought there'd be a moment to breathe
I turned around to find
all our other children
waiting for their small taste of presence
of recognition
reprieve

I've waited months this year for reprieve
but the cycle is deep
the learnings are full
and the focus or message
I think I'm searching for
is probably not the pathway
but an alleyway of interest
walking, dancing,
holding myself
in these alleyways
to unknown destinations

dr veronica moule

bits and pieces

what is the role of the pregnant woman
in these days of medicalisation
reductionism
this illusion…delusion
that we can divide up all aspects of woman
into blood pressure and blood glucose
vitamin supplements
ultrasound monitoring
if all her 'bits and pieces' are right
then she'll be OK

so, women watch their 'bits and pieces'
trying to be good
do the right thing
and somewhere in those bits and pieces
the whole can get lost
the wonder
the fluidity of change
the expansion and opening
the miracle of the coming child
of course, we know a child is coming
who says they need parenting by the state before they arrive?

it's the pregnant woman who holds this child
let's leave her in the wonder of this holding
place the medicine in its medicine box
invite woman to float in the abyss
the miracle forming within
the role of the pregnant woman
is to be steeped in the wonder

to allow it to move her
from the rhythm of her depths
she can listen to her body
feel it opening
find the pathway she'll travel
as she unravels herself
to allow her child to emerge

broader

I'm pumped
a little uncontainable
opportunity knocks
and I'm barrelling through
with this big, bold, broad vision
of a simple, normal,
ridiculously typical idea

lay myself open
passionate
capable
driven
uncompromising
small steps towards a successful model
from a successful model
with broader breath
and broader depth

and the decision maker is unclear
we need to find the way
for us, the clinicians
guided by the women
to be the decision-makers
we can accept their parameters
policy pieces of paper
if it allows us the breath
the depth
allows our knowing to sing and shine
and bathe in glorious birth

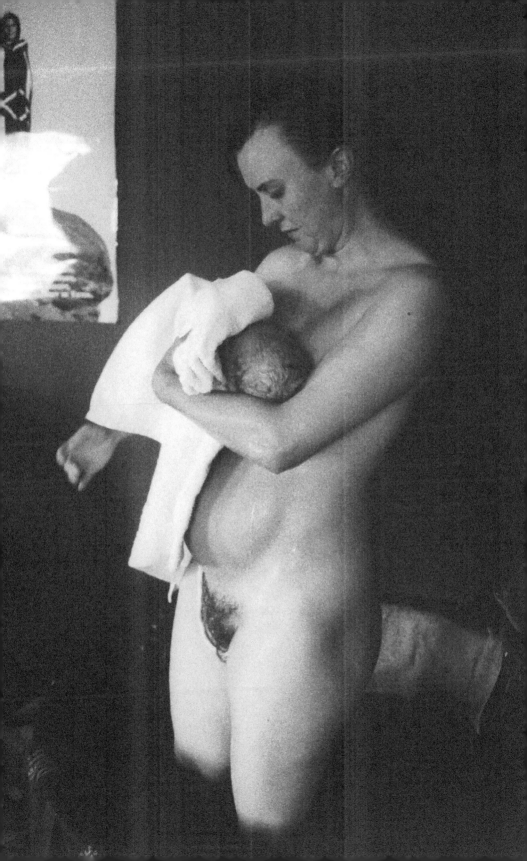

Hades

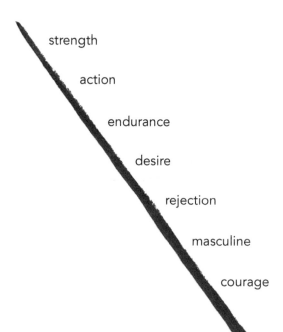

strength

action

endurance

desire

rejection

masculine

courage

courage

I am woman
trying to unravel culture
ridiculous societal rules
...lie down to birth
be quiet
be obedient...

actually
hold me how I want to be held
or don't hold me at all
I come
with all my wounds
to navigate myself
all my raw potency
calling me from my depths

I have courage
to stand in my strength
in honour of myself

I have courage
beyond my own knowing
I hold the inner power of birthing woman

Artemis to Kali

Artemis
strengthen my body for the fight
muscle bound, fit, ready for action
movement, endurance and breath
bold woman
your eyes are clear, your arrow straight

but Kali
I'm twisting and turning
and drawn
deeply, powerfully, irrationally

she's not listening to the voice of reason
she's searching for opportunities
seductive predator
how do I chaperone my life from her embrace

but…she is the birthing energy
the chaos
the transition
the step to open-ness and wisdom
surrender…

dr veronica moule

solace

at times of stress
I go for solace
travelling deep within myself
looking for my breath
looking for stillness
riding the waves of chaos
warrior woman
on my solo journey

and I've tried to free this
this need to pull down my barrier
disconnect from the world
as I search for solace within
my children have been my bridge
my freedom to cry with them
to ask to be held

and the pattern has shifted
when they search for support
at their times of stress
they can ask that of us
not just holding a dependence on self

and I'm proud of this change
some things can shift within a generation
I wonder if they can shift in me in this lifetime

be gone

you do not belong
in the depths of woman
and woman calls clearly
I have suffered abuse
I have birthed my child
my placenta is not ready
in your time frame

she asks for the young woman doctor
to be the hand
not the old obstetrician man
and we honoured that request
young woman
doing the job of patriarchy

my hand glided
between placenta and womb
like cupping soft wet sand at the water's edge
placenta was scooped
and released
and her uterus called
be gone
constricting
pushing my hand out
shutting the cervix
like bolting a door
you do not belong in here
in the depths of this woman

dr veronica moule

she wasn't bleeding
what right did we have
to tell her when to birth her placenta
we have equipment to fix problems
but we're not equipped to wait for the problem
the problem that might not come
invading her body for our own fear
of blood
of time frames and judgements

roar

labour song
stripped bare and raw
rises from her depths

labour song deepening
as her baby descends
through the depths of her pelvis
and she roars with her opening
surrendering

it's not an empty roar
we know what we're roaring for
release the shackles of patriarchy
the cultural constructs
we're stepping into our capacity as woman
the world of woman
in all her raw complexity
beyond anything man can know
to the depths of her cellular level
to the symphony of her hormones
awe inspiring
Roar of the wild birthing woman

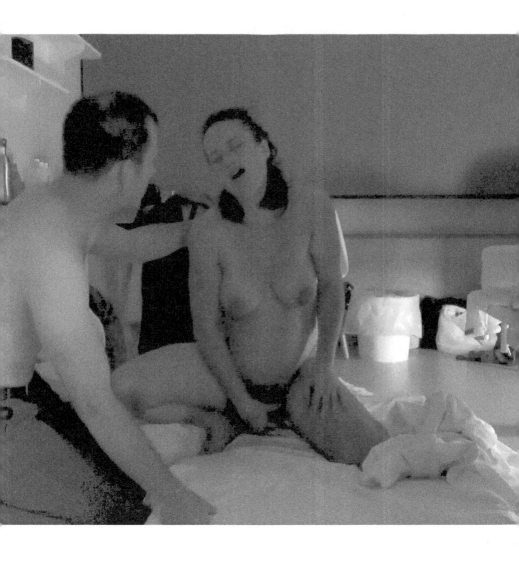

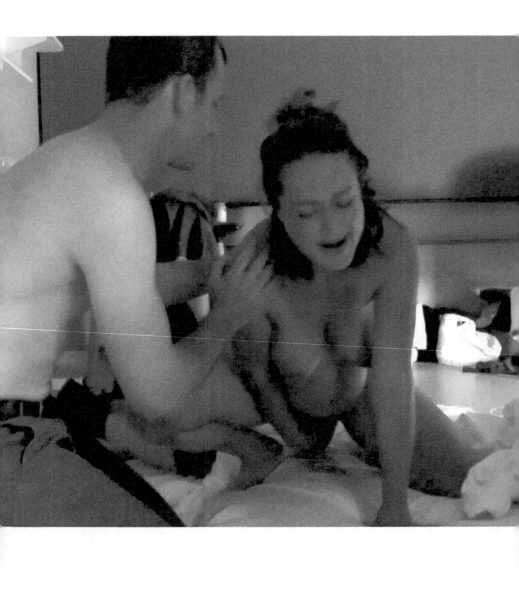

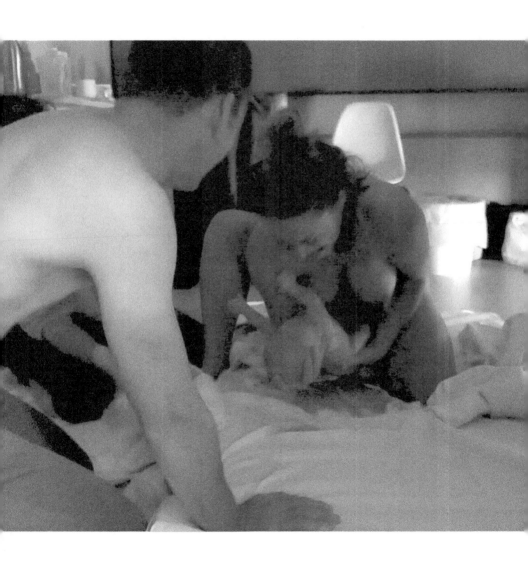

Kore

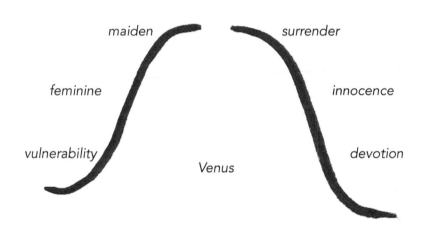

maiden   surrender

feminine   innocence

vulnerability   devotion

Venus

stage fright

...the 3rd stage, birth of the placenta...

who are you?
holding tight, constricting
until there'll be no breath left
gasping for embodiment

rational, distant power
disinterested in the beauty,
in striving for maternal capacity / capability / depth

in the beginning
there was mother and baby
the 2 as one, becoming the 2
then breathing into each other
touching, searching for their dance together
finding a way back to oneness

why interrupt?
who says the guide should become the block,
the barrier, the inhibitor of the space

sacred space
trespassing

dance

overwhelm
arriving vulnerable
ready for diving into the depths
then people
many, many people
overwhelm
Artemis came, watchful
strength warrior
she's not vulnerable
she's also not the guidance I was expecting
or wanting
my community holds me in the dance
I can breathe and find myself
flow my tears
roar my pains
but this is busy and full
faces are here
but not the space for holding
for intimacy
for dancing release
I need to hold myself in this space
like my 5 year old has held me
and be held by the music
close your eyes...be with the music
I dance my depths
more broadly
into catharsis
in connection
in my community

dr veronica moule

my dance floor midwives
are not strangers in the moment
my continuity of carers
community care
helping me traverse my depths

tears

tears and tears
as I reach back to my 5 year old
and see her strength
her courage
feel her, with love
I am bold and capable and uncompromising
and passionate and committed
and I love all these things about me
which is different to loving me
what is my capacity
with my abandoned loves
who question my presence
maybe, I need to love myself
and thank myself for loving myself

this year I've shown myself love
through service
in nourishing my body
through words
in poetry
through touch
with love and lust
now through gift giving
the gift of the dance
many ways to show love
and the little girl opens her heart
to find space to receive love
from myself
and the tears flow

dr veronica moule

surrender

vulnerable
again
maybe this is the sisterhood link
I'm unpractised at sisterly togetherness
so the wounds cut
the wounds of exclusion
of lack of recognition
of being unimportant or not seen
in this place where I give my all
and meet my all

mentoring change
will be about letting go
waves of presence and absence
responsibility and freedom
today there were moments in labour and birth
of holding woman to a depth of breath
of calm
of knowing
reconnecting her to the moment in her last birth,
her first birth
my hands again in the same position
bringing her back to the moment she shifted
to allowing, surrender, trust
knowing of her body
the thread of continuity guiding woman from birth to birth
and mothering between
each birth imprints
child, let's revisit your birthplace
the place your mother surrendered herself
to allow you to emerge

maybe I need to surrender myself
to allow a rebirthing of our birthing service
but it will come in waves
of presence and breath
of release and allowing
growing a new child from birth to maturity
waves of vulnerability and loss
as my fertility will wane
and the wise crone will emerge
as guide over warrior

dr veronica moule

loss

we didn't know
we didn't know that the pause
those few hours of stillness
was when most of you became absent

we didn't know through the depths of labour
until the tide turned
the time to descend
and it all became too much
the skerrick of hanging on
was pushed over the edge

we didn't know that two days before
was your moment, your turning point
when you released vast pools of meconium
that flowed through your world
stained your skin, your cord, your placenta
and sank to the depths of your lungs
ebbed and flowed there

your tide had turned
and when the call of labour asked a little more of you
the little more that was too much
when your absence was complete
despite our desperate calls to bring you back
when your eyes had gone...

we can force in breath
and we can pump blood for you
but we can't bring back life
to eyes that have already left

learnings

what do we do
when we stretch and open ourselves
make room in our lives, in ourselves for another
for being more than we've been

what do we do
when that space we have opened isn't filled
when the wanting is not satisfied
when the space is empty
when who we have opened for and waited for doesn't stay
doesn't survive this great transition
from in-utero to air
comes without breath
comes without life

what do we do
when we are witness to this pain
when our job is to hold
to be clinically capable
to be compassionate and gentle
how do we hold ourselves
when we are holding the parents
how do we hold ourselves, and find our breath
receive the reflections of our actions
learning of our abilities
whilst sitting in judgement of our lessons
how do we bring compassion, kindness to ourselves
to not run away from our pain
to find our breath in the learnings
to grieve this experience to its completion

dr veronica moule

can we see that we have also opened ourselves
made ourselves a little bigger
found a space within ourselves
that is filled with both grief and experience
learnings for our hands to hold,
our hearts to hold
so we can hold others with more wisdom
if we're called to do this again

vagina

can I put evening primrose oil in my vagina?
I've heard it's great for labour
you can put whatever you want in your vagina – it's your vagina
this sounds like the raspberry leaf tea story – 'great for labour'
you can have as many cups of tea as you like

but, when you've journeyed through labour,
and opened your body
and pushed out your baby,
then you deserve the glory for that
and you should hold the glory
my feminist is offended that the cup of tea is the hero
when the hero is always the birthing woman

what is it
that denies women the voice,
the recognition
the glory
what makes the dad the hero for being there
or cutting a cord with a pair of scissors
or the taxi driver the hero

I've felt a potency this year
way beyond the patriarchal rules and structure
a big, bold and uncontained potency
the world would be very different
if we women all walked in our potency
felt our potency
and could communicate our potencies

dr veronica moule

and we would laugh with deep knowing
about the ridiculousness
of what a cup of tea can bring
to the enduring, unfolding, surrendering wild woman ride of labour

beyond

take your breath deep into your pelvis
breathe into the muscles around your bottom, your vagina
and let them soften

breathe deeply
into the muscles of your pelvis
let them soften
make the pathway for your baby a little easier

take your breath deep into your pelvis
meet this contraction
let it be a little bigger
beyond your breath
beyond the structure you know as yourself
beyond your holding
beyond the light
just a little bit further
into the release of yourself
past the peak
let yourself be a little softer
as this wave comes
you will wash to the other side
back to your breath
breathe
softness
and rest

dr veronica moule

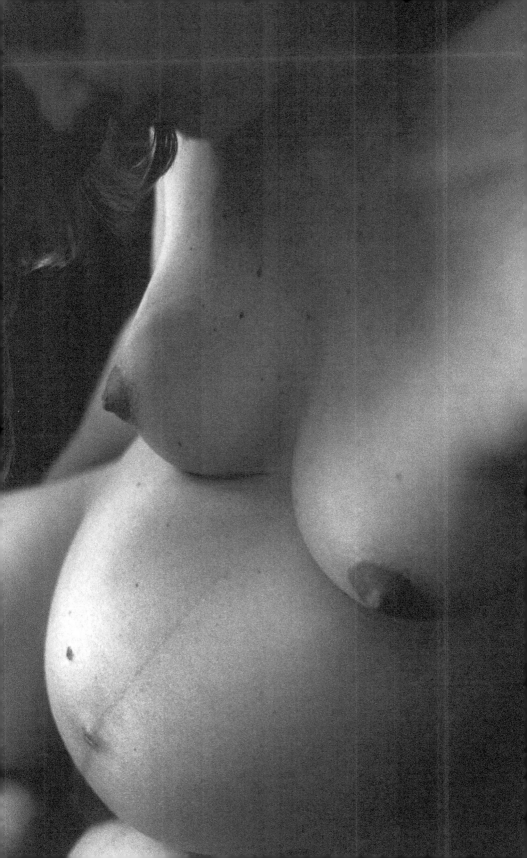

Light

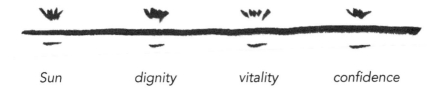

Sun   dignity   vitality   confidence

burning

the burning
stretching heat
just before baby is born

hot towels now!
we meet heat with heat
we're not trying to cool this fire
burning our way into motherhood

burning beyond belief
we are beyond culture
at the precipice of time
in a moment
everything will change
nothing will be the same again

woman on fire
releasing her child

pause

pause
when breath is slow and deep and rich
the feeling of pause
at both in-breath and post out-breath

it's not patience
as patience suggests waiting
in suppressed anticipation of what's next

pause in stillness
maybe I'm finding a moment
my moment of stillness for this year

dr veronica moule

bearing witness

it's a wild dance
running, breathing, rowing, singing
my way through boundless space
shedding my protective insulation
exposing my layers –
dark and light and multi-coloured
peeling my way within and without
swirling, directionless
other than away from the boundaries of patriarchy
to a place where I can turn and see its flavours –
the borders and boundaries, the rules
held regardless of reason or fact
the linear time structure

I am a broad landscape
a tree may look to be a signpost
as is the earth walked on to get there
and the creek that flows its own winding way
but not the fence posts
and not the straining wire
I turn into a kangaroo
jumping them with humorous disrespect
I saw a joey hurry into her mother's pouch yesterday
in a convoluted jumble
movement and maternal protection is chaotic and effective

I usually play the role of guide
I am now learning about others bearing witness
and you have been thrillingly surprised that I'm sharing

and probably surprised at the depth of the sharing
receiving witness feels like sheltering for breath in the trees
whilst I walk and dance and sing the earth between

dr veronica moule

birthing tree

sturdy
grounded
soft
gentle
quiet
holding
holding earth
holding air

central cavity
with inner folds
ledges for squatting support
birthing coming from within
completed
within mother nature's holding
home
womb
doorway entrance like vulval folds
rugged exterior
fired charcoal inner walls
smooth folds on entry
smooth inner folds at windows
small passageways out
if I was to birth on land
not under the sea
I could find my breath
and open my body
within the inner walls
of this tree

I stood in thanks
in reverence
my hands held together
at my heart
and I'm mirroring the tree
2 sturdy hands like the trunk
inner cavity
a tree of reverence

dr veronica moule

mandala

mandala
installation
bits and pieces
my courage
my integrity
my ferocious oxytocin fuelled wild woman
my passion
my commitment
my bits and pieces
gather them up
spread them around
circular patterns
patterns of recognition
patterns of behaviour
but the dance flows within and around
circuiting
and we gather more capacity
layers and layers
searching for a bigger whole

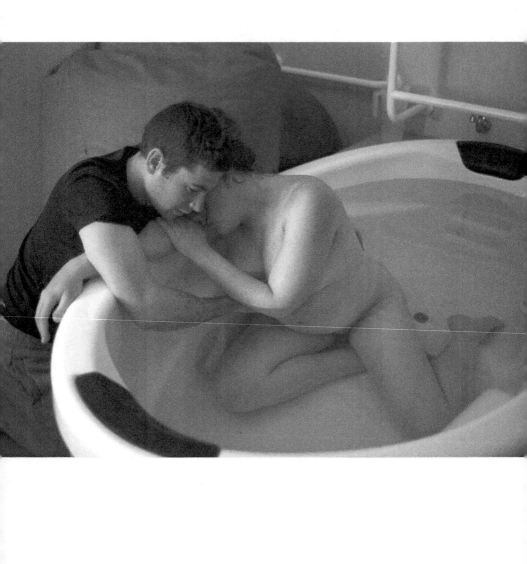

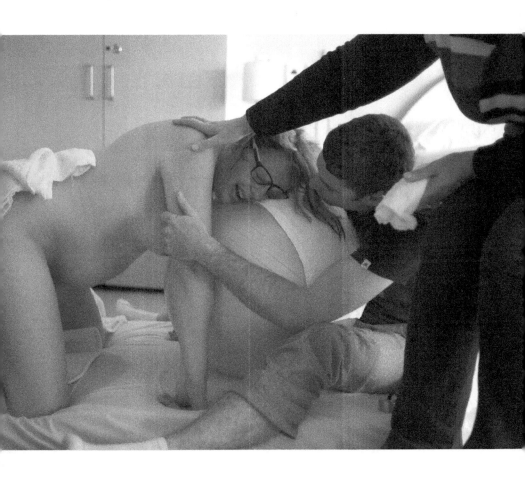

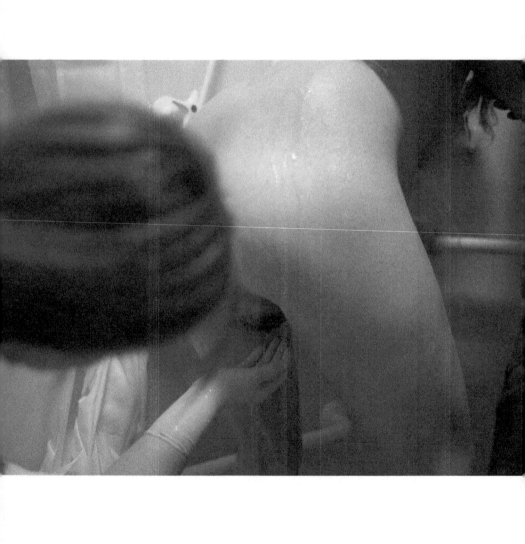

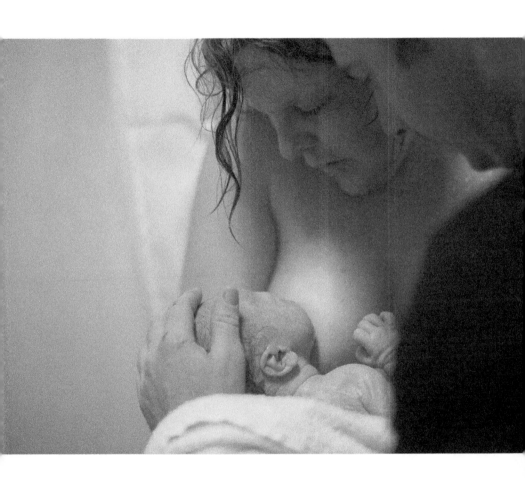

Persephone

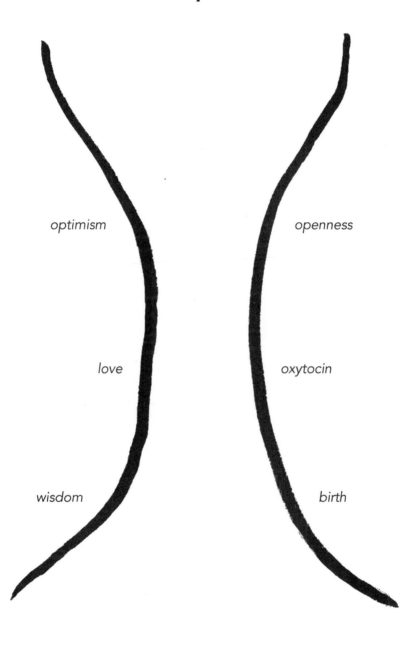

optimism   openness

love   oxytocin

wisdom   birth

Persephone

we think of the maiden as naïve
accidentally noshing – she has tasted the dark
now she is captured forever
to cycle through the underworld as Persephone

she returns to the light
she returns from the dark recesses of herself
she's embodied them in her flesh
the pomegranate
ovarian fruit

the Greek myth
written as though woman wouldn't want to know the dark
embody the dark
carry the wisdom of the underworld
with her into the light

yet all women do
we cycle
through our blood
then our lightness
through desire
through the disconnect
the internal musings
the moody stretches
as we try and pretend we're 'as usual'
but we're cycling into the dark
in preparation to bleed again
it is what we do monthly
this menstrual preparation
for the grand extravaganza
of labour and birth

embodied

we hugged goodbye,
my first son, nearing 21
and heading into manhood
the tears flowed for us both
and as I held him,
I could feel myself holding him as I did when he was a baby

I danced that night,
a dance that opens me and shows me my inner self
and pouring from me into the dance
was the dance we danced when he was a baby
21 years that dance,
our dance, as the dance differed with each child
sat in my body
embodied

birthing politics and patriarchy have hammered me this year
responsibility, accountability
stand up, prove yourself

my feminine calls
paddling the lake, I'm drawn to the house where my 2 youngest
were born
driving to the coast, I'm drawn down the road to Glenlyon,
where my 2nd child was born
I need to go to Modewarre,
birthplace of my first child
birthplace of myself as mother

dr veronica moule

the birthing place
birthing on country
birthing where I live and raise my family
turn the soil, plant the trees, the placenta,
breathe in the land
the rhythm of the seasons
and the rhythm of labour and birth

throw your policies and structures at me
my feminist can see you
and she draws on the earth, mother earth, my birthing earth
reconnects me to my source
embodied in birth, in dance, in place

breath in the third stage

breathe
breathing your baby out into the world
with gentleness
the mother's embrace
the meeting, the wonder
the mystery both ending and beginning
who is this child, who has come to join the family

this is the space of the breath
the newborn, learning a new skill in breathing,
the mother, breathing in her child

when my 4th child was born, as with my other 3,
I held him, and breathed him into me
the sweet smell of a newborn baby,
and their out breath
smelling as pure as rainforest air
with every breath I took,
nuzzling and smelling him
I could feel my uterus contract
my knowing uterus
deep, powerful, healing contractions
clenching my uterus
from smelling and breathing my newborn
primitive pathways
nature's wisdom
imprint my child into my brain through smell,
through breath
my hormones
penetrating my blood brain barrier

dr veronica moule

my oxytocin
peak love
peak capacity and internal strength

together we shared in the breath
in – in – in – in - …. out
in – in – in – in - …. out
oxytocin breathing, breathing in love…

who is this institution
whose agenda is it
to break the primitive bond
to prevent, to block
all the love flowing between mother and baby

this is the moment
it is a complete hormonal experience
the woman who birthed her baby wants this
she knows that the wonder of birth comes from within her
she can open her body…
she can push or breathe her baby out
she can hold her baby in nature's hormonal embrace
and as she breathes her baby in, her uterus contracts
efficient, strong uteruses excel in contracting

tired, exhausted uteruses may well need help
let's not compromise women with efficient uteruses
by giving artificial oxytocin
for the sake of other people's agendas

man-waves

'this is the best feeling
it comes in waves
it's overwhelming
washing over me
too much, I need to steady
then another wave comes'

says young man, wide eyed
at the birth of his first child

he tells the story of oxytocin
the surging peaks
the rest between
this young man
speaking the words few notice or share
this man who stretched himself
in his youth
stretched his boundaries
until they had no walls
neurotransmitter explosion
of abundance and depletion
over and over

he's felt the expanse
the initiation of peyote
without the grounding of community ritual
held by loose threads
with others, barely tethered

dr veronica moule

and now he is held in futures family
with woman and child
he feels nature's ecstasy
and can give words
to the wonder of the neurotransmitters

womb

journey to the wild depths of motherhood
I breathed, embraced,
held you within my womb
not held with hands
that may squeeze or loosen their grip
held you with every organ of my body
caressed you with my pain as I laboured and you birthed
then held you in gentleness
in my arms
in my heart
in the depth of our inspiration and release of breath

then life, motherhood
multitasking
compartmentalising
chop me up in little bits
and scatter me around
like seeds to the earth
hoping for germination

then a moment comes
a moment of illness
that strips away the detail, the multitasking,
the busyness of daily life
and leaves me raw, open
with vision of what's important
and spirals, funnels that energy
into being
into presence
into the togetherness of the womb

dr veronica moule

unconditional love
calling me back
into the wild birthing depths of motherhood
where there is only the moment
only presence
togetherness

rebirthing

and Kali came
into the dance
with soft gentleness
who would have thought
she could be gentle
wicked trickery?
and the dance became bold
and Kali called in her strength
moved me
flowing Kali through me
of me
me

the wind picked up
cooling draft
I am a bird
lifted by the breeze
lifted up in lightness
soaring
gliding
turning

my feet ground themselves
I am the sheoak
the breeze blows through me
making me sing
sturdier
I am the message tree
my branches crossed
waving in the breeze
my trunk

dr veronica moule

sunk deep in mother earth
now I am the birthing tree
I am in the birthing tree
labouring
labour song moves me
opens me
centres me
I am birthing
opening, releasing
I am birthing … myself…

all year I've felt this birthing process
gestation
chaos
transition
never knowing what I was birthing
I thought I was birthing our new birthing service
but it was me
I birthed myself
then held myself
in my own loving touch…
tenderness
infant girl
toddler girl
5 year old girl
re-exploring my re-birthed self

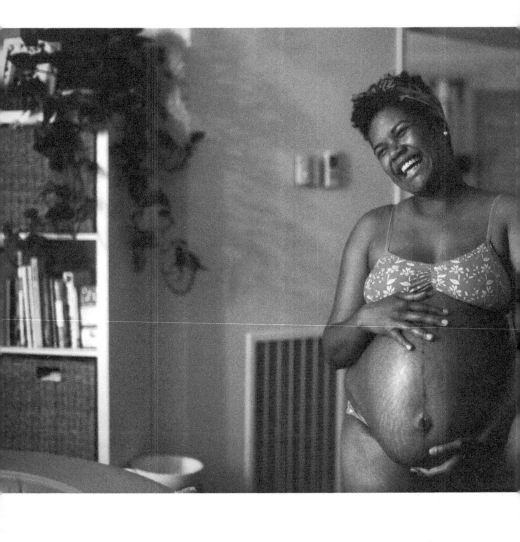

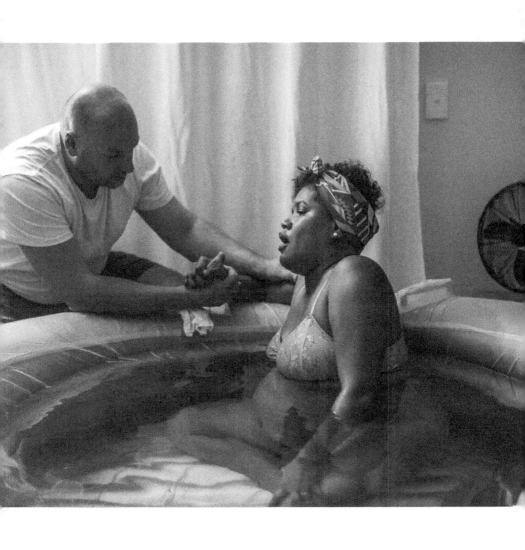

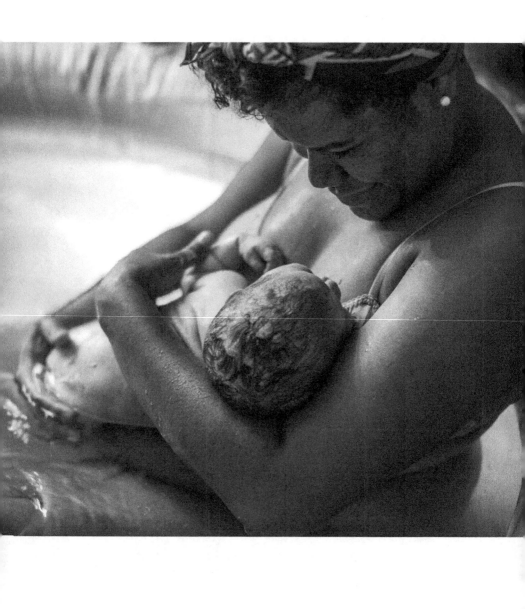

Embodied midwifery

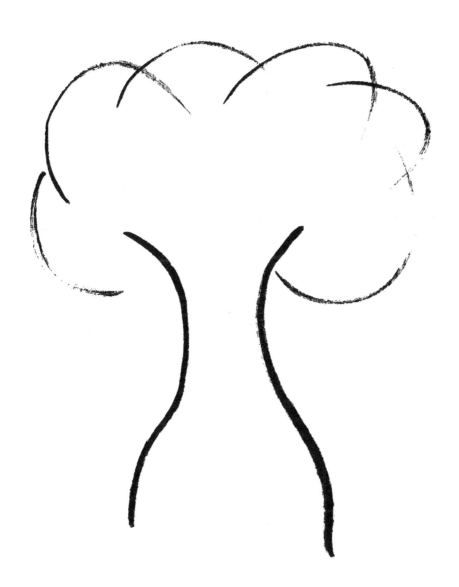

physiological guide

how do we guide women in labour
not sit in observation, judgement, analysis
or tell them how to be

how do we invite women
into their unravelling
into surrender
take their breath
into the depths of themselves
release the tension in their muscles
reduce the restriction in their bodies
help their baby move down

how do we help women
be at one with this enormous process
invite women to not hold it back
nor try and push it forwards
to sit in the space of the wonder
listening to the unfolding of their bodies
to be present with their body opening
and their child being born

can we listen to our own physiology
can we breathe deeply into our bodies
release the tension in our muscles
reduce the restriction in our bodies
how do we stop getting caught in risk-aversion
tightening up our bodies
how do we heal our wounds
from past complicated births
integrate the experience
into a knowing in our hands
not a restriction in our hearts

allowing

what are we doing as birth-workers
if we're not 'doing'
if we are allowing
if we are the leaning post
the safe space
the nurturer who gives a woman permission to trust herself
to let go

if we were to see ourselves as healers
rather than mechanics
if we were willing to allow ourselves to be stretched
to a place of discomfort
because that's what this individual woman needs

to know the spaces of normal
to be capable of intervening in the abnormal
yet be aware that there is a great zone in between
and that this is the space to allow breath
to allow ourselves to be stretched
to be willing to be wrong
to learn
to be forever students in this mystery of birth

dr veronica moule

i am a midwife

I am a midwife,
although that is not the title I carry
I am a midwife
because I will advocate for you in birth
to the depths of my being
from the depths of my being
to the depths of where I desired advocacy
when it was my body
my inner woman
labouring and birthing
if that is the depth that you wish to travel

yes, I will advocate for you
to the depths of your choice
with clarity and breathe
with shining light on darkness
darkness that may be steering you into unnecessarily stormy
waters

calm
breathe
embodied
I am a midwife

oxytocin

am I addicted to oxytocin?
this wondrous hormone
that spreads my breath throughout my chest
and opens my mind in lightness and dark
boundless connection of self to universe

the cycles and spikes
peaks from attending births
lasting 3 days
coming regularly yet irregularly

from the depths of wonder of my birthing
4 times peaked
each held in quiet sanctuary
deep in mystical physiology
and breastfeeding
14 years of satisfaction in my breasts
sometimes I needed to breastfeed
to fall back asleep
like a post-coital release and sleep

and that's where this question arises
someone tried to take away my post-birthing peak
challenge the physiology
and birthing numbers are down
my body is hungry
demanding, wanting
take me to the oxytocin moment
cycle me there again and again
to the sanctuary before breath
to presence with the boundless universe

dr veronica moule

receiving

I need to be held
in this birthing process
birthing something within or without me
clarity yet to arrive
that was the message in the dance
I need to be held
it's not time for the boldly independent birthing woman
I need to receive my midwives

and the hospital judgements feel harsh
and naïve
I'm not being seen for who I am
it's not a competition
why is this precision
in breath, in presence
so hard to understand
embodiment, responsibility
intertwining together

we did lock eyes, birthing woman and I
2 minutes after the birth, on my arrival
2 connected women
in a crash scene
and she was ok
in a 'fuck, this crazy thing just happened,
isn't it ridiculous' kind of way
and I wanted more for her
I wanted her to experience being held in presence and breath
but she's ok
there's not much to debrief

and what there is
she does with eyebrows raised and a smirk
she got a typical, panicked, usual birth
her fight came later, with donor milk

and I received an astonishing awareness
driving down the hill, 2 minutes before arriving
the pure smell of amniotic fluid, flooded me
the knowing, at the moment of birth
transmitted through me
captured, or released, in smell

dr veronica moule

intimacy

what is intimacy?
open-hearted connection
breathing together
trust
opening ourselves, our inner being
to share with another

my work is intimate
I breathe with people
they navigate their emotional selves
women open their bodies in birth
surrender themselves
in my trusting hands
and as they do that
my body opens
my uterus contracts
I know how deeply a woman is in labour
by listening to my own body
this is a deep intimacy
and the intimacy I share with women in birth
progresses to intimate friendships
open-hearted, honest, soul-searching, free, fun

there is a boundlessness in these relationships
we have embodied each other,
our experiences together
this embodiment comes from breath and trust
it is a spiritual connection between women
it is boundless, because it can only occur without boundaries
this is part of my joy and my calling to work in birthing
birthing feels like my spiritual journey

aching womb

my womb ached today
contracting in unison
with a woman, deep in labour

I sat in my breath
a little unsure in my mind
if the baby would be ok
as she hadn't had any ultrasounds
but I felt settled and OK in my body

it is more wondrous
almost too painful to watch
seeing mother and child connect
when so recently
I've witnessed the opposite
witnessed and felt the desperate yearning of loss

and I wonder now
if my womb contracting was trying to squeeze out the recent pain
cleansing me to my organic depths
searching through my wanting
as I grieve for the family, for the stillborn child
and as I write this
I can again feel my contracting womb

maybe our wombs are organs of grief
as well as organs of accommodation,
nurturing, nourishment
organs of love

dr veronica moule

legacy

Kali's depths descend
and release
into the lady of the lake
and who is she?
floating in the amniotic waters
foetal and maternal
nurtured and held
in a warm watery embrace

I'm embracing legacy
we stand in strength
in normal, capable
I'm looking for expansion, extension
let's extend beyond our current hold
into the boundless space
of woman
of birth
through the waters of holding
of woman-song
harmonic waters
reflected
embraced
engulfed
into surrender

I felt lost in my watery realm
then my fire returned
determined
uncompromising
fire and water

creates warm water for birthing
earth and fire
carry me in strength
to gently, persuasively fight
for women
for midwives
for the legacy of beautiful birthing

dr veronica moule

midwifery

being with-woman
this is more than physical presence –
more than touch
more than seeing the unnecessary structures and rules
and fighting against these
or dancing around them

there is an emotional presence
an open-hearted caring
empathy of her past travels –
her traumas and heartaches
her triumphs and vulnerabilities
being with her emotionally
as this journey of labour
rips open her defences
and lays her emotionally bare
awaiting the moment
to be filled emotionally
with the devastatingly deep love
a mother can have
after opening her body and releasing her child

there is an embodied spiritual presence
that we as midwives have with birthing women
this exists, whether conscious or not
and is a deeply powerful energy
if brought to the midwives' consciousness
it may be the energy that shifts 2 women from friendly strangers
to deep soul and spirit wanderers together
in the maze of the weird human world

when we midwife on all 3 levels,
our inner woman carries that patriarchal box of rules and
    regulations
many fundamentally useful
to ensure the physical safety of woman and child
we do need to meet obstacles with a plan
our first role, security on the physical plane

embodied midwifery
allowing our breath to navigate
the innate knowing between women
like the housemates' menstrual cycles aligning
women are connected beyond consciousness...

in my final year of med school
a year of very intensive study and togetherness
my study partner was pregnant
and through that year
my belly developed a linea nigra
the dark pigment line on a pregnant belly
the hormones required for a linea nigra
are expressed at the hypothalamus
my body and hers were communicating
from somewhere higher than the hypothalamus

we know we meet in birth on a hormonal level
the oxytocin high
there is intimacy and love that flows
between women and birth attendant
the endorphin rush
that floats us away with a knowing smile that lasts for days

embodied midwifery
taking our breath into our depths
and feeling the opening that's happening
in our bodies

dr veronica moule

feeling our uterus contract
feeling the muscles of our pelvic floor
their tightness and their weakness
feeling our backs
the strength and dysfunction in our spines,
our sacrum stretching and opening
the pressure feelings in our bowels as the baby descends
taking our breath into these parts of ourselves
feeling the change the breath offers
feeling the changes in our own bodies
as the woman progresses in her labour

sometimes labour and birth call us to action
we do embody actions and capabilities
in our hands
in our minds
in our hearts
and in our embodied spiritual beings
we can open the patriarchal box of tricks
gather the required skills
and still stand with the inner woman in command...

we can respond to crisis from our heart space
my inner woman surging
pouring my strength, myself into the woman, the baby
and later when we meet
there is a love-like knowing that sits between and around us
together we navigated life's biggest challenge
and came through with breath
and wonder
and thankfulness
patriarchy thinks it's the all-knowing rescuer
but we know that we can do those tricks
and be-with as well

and this story I'm writing to midwives
there is a depth to our midwifery
a depth beyond comprehension
but a depth that we can bring to consciousness
and maybe together
if we share our consciousness of these depths
we can bring deep wisdom to our inner women
that will circle around to other women in our care

dr veronica moule

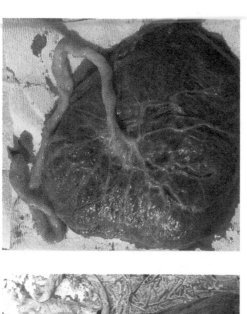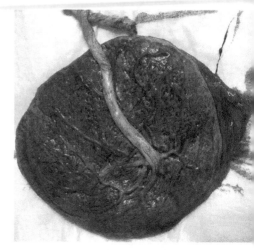

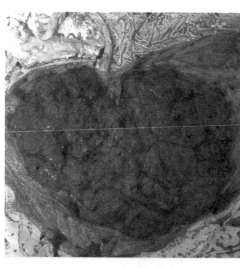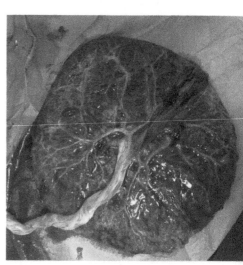

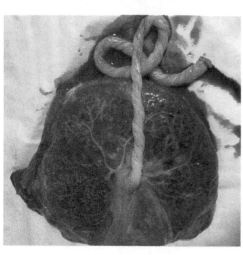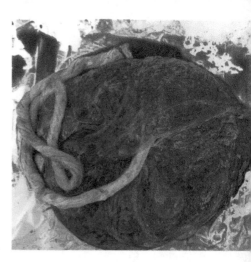

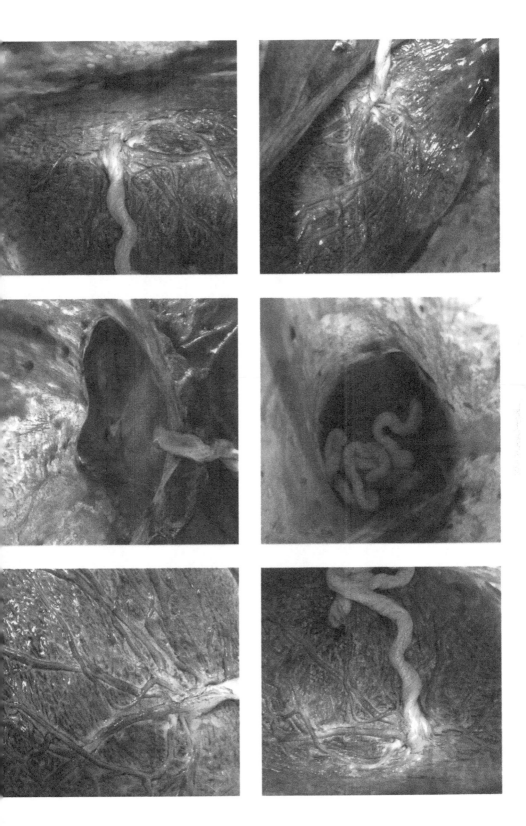

birth stories of
my children

Jarah

Aidan

Callum

Ben

Jarah

damp awakening...clear fluid trickles...dozing between irregular
tightenings...mind preparing for early start
walking ...pause...birds singing...trees swaying...
cows feeding...pause...warm sun...soft breeze...walking
white horses shining in the bush...silhouette...family...
peaceful exuberance...walking

pink liquor dripping...breathe...cervix opening...
hay bales supporting squat...focus earth...breathe
'good contractions' says my intrinsic midwife...fast...regular...
call Phil home...breathe
water...warm and buoyant...immediate intense contractions...
accelerating opening

back pains...sacrum throbbing...need firm pressure...beautiful
deep pelvic vocalising...focus sacrum...I hear myself
pushing...call Patrice
back pains...coccyx...more heat!!!...pelvis opening...I feel my
baby's head...deep loud vocalising...pushing

anal pressure...intense anal pressure...I can't fit a baby out my
anus...aargh...breathe
stretching perineum...everything feels tight...quiet
contractions...focus breathing...focus perineum

all is calm between contractions...quiet...cool of evening...soft
peace
quiet pushing...baby moving, kicking, pushing – helping...more
head out...stretching perineum
quiet pushing, panting...breathe, breathe, breathe...head is born...

*I see my baby's head between my legs...my hands caress my
    baby's beautiful hairy head
pushing...pushing...babe leaves my body...into the water...
    surfacing*

*my baby is born...
welcome my love
from the quiet of your birth
we welcome your beautiful song and dance
active, alert and aware
miraculous birth of my baby Jarah
wondrous birth of myself as woman, as mother*

Aidan

spiritual birth, can it be
when safety is in the clinical, physical
with separatist acknowledgement of the emotional
is it misunderstanding of the spirit?

spirit – the essence of new life
the bond that weaves through the waves of labouring women
continent to continent
moment to moment
women labouring and birthing
disconnected in space
malnourished emotionally

where is the keeper of the sacred-space
the wise woman spirit watching, being
knowing the process
understanding the space
protector from the spirit world

why can I find people
women
who want to control or begrudge the space
why can't I find somebody to just be
to revel in the experience of birth
to share the intensity, the passion, the joy
to alleviate the pain of the search, the sadness
I have sadness
overwhelming sadness
sadness that I haven't found someone to share the joy
and protect the space from desires to control
misaligned duties

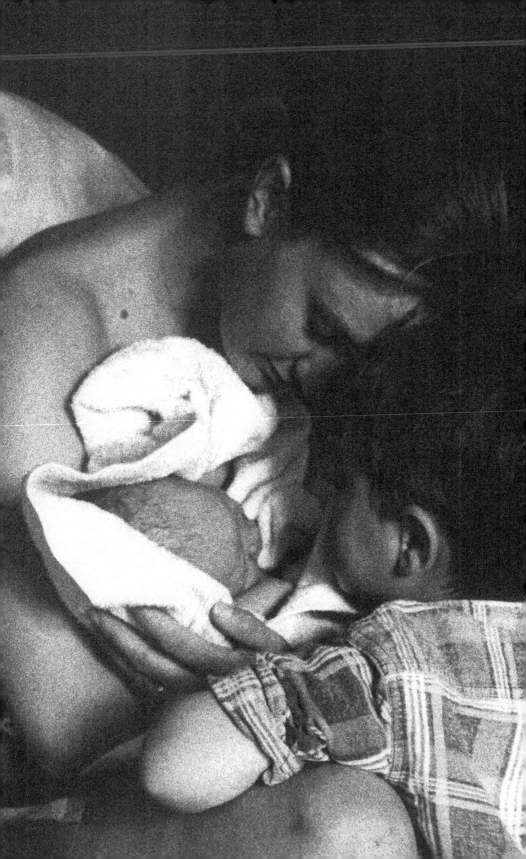

Callum

summer Solstice 2002
standing on the bluestone
to connect with the moon
earth, rock, woman, babe, Luna tricks

the westerly wind blew and blew
the wind howled through the trees
as I howled on my knees
in the warmth of the bath
the night was wild and peaceful and calm
by candlelight in the corner of our bedroom

Jarah and Aidan slept through the roars
as my body opened, until your head was released
when Jarah joined us in body
Aidan joined us in sleep
and Callum you arrived, birthed, entered a new world

magical boy, cheeky and fun
determined, self-assured adventurous Callum
you bring more lightness and brightness to our family

Ben

he came in song
meditative cleansing
of the walls of my womb
as the cello, the bells
reverberated my body
then her voice
rising through her bare feet
from the earth
from her depths
rising through her body
then it rose through mine
through my cleansed uterus
and sang down my fallopian tubes
come ovum
your time to sing has come
we conceived that night
in the presence of song

women gathered to bless this child
led by gentle midwife choir-mistress
we sang together
birthing songs
women's songs
welcoming songs
singing this child into the world

dr veronica moule

as this child grows
he falls into song
everyday
exploding from him
and gently oozing from him
spontaneous
creatively changing words
and singing-along
our son is of and from song

dawn

we greeted dawn with a twinge and a splash
dawn of a new day
a day without time
a day of change
the greatest change of my life on this day
of orange-pink skies and welcoming bird songs

rhythm and flow
heat and pain
walking and screaming
open heart
open mind
open body
I open my life to a new person, a new soul

there's a moment when two souls meet
a moment free of time
a moment of magic
my memory lingers on that sweet moment
following a day of work
of rhythm and pain
of walking, screaming
awaiting the moment

dr veronica moule

the backyard looks different now
it is a place to walk with the rhythm and flow
with the heat and pain
the bath looks different now
water for buoyancy and comfort
flowing water
easing the pain
the bath of my most sacred act
the bath of birthing
and now the bath of bathing,
of a joyful child's screams
of breastfeeding
flowing warm water
always there to reconnect me with the moment,
with timelessness
with sacredness

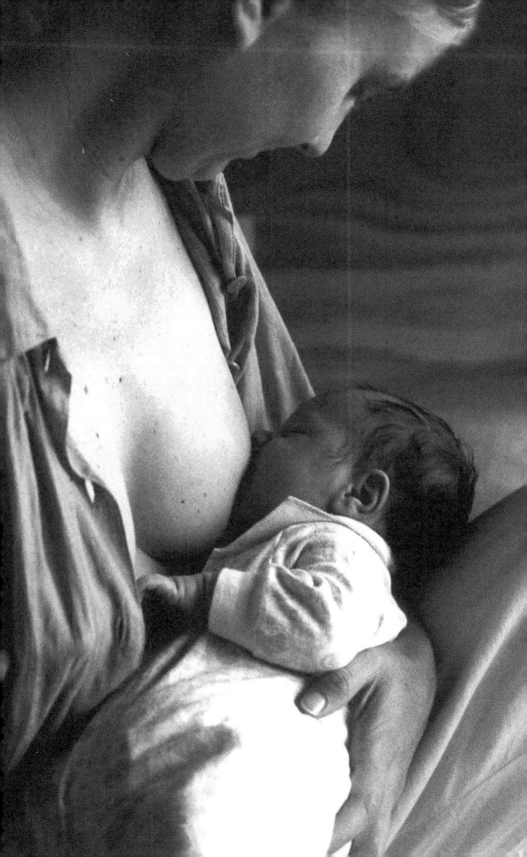

acknowledgements

to my sons Jarah, Aidan, Callum and Ben, through whom I have experienced the astonishing wonder of birth and unconditional love, and who continue to show me how to be a mother, in their own individual ways

to Phil for our love, for this amazing journey we share in our relationship, and your commitment to parenting that has held our family when the chaos of birthing calls

to my women friends, who held me and walked beside me as I unravelled and reformed to be more of my authentic self, with special thanks to Arabella Davison, Samantha Ward, Louisa Hope, Marg Peck, Marie Louise Lapeyre and Sky Simpson

to the Castlemaine 5 rhythms dance community, for the safety of the space and witnessing my journeying, with special thanks to Thais Sansom, Meredith Davies and David Juriansz, and all who meet me on the dance floor

to the artistry that has brought beauty beyond words, thanks to Denise Martin, Zoe Amor, Phoebe Barton, Katie Varallo, Lil Pearce, Amanda Bourdon, Rusila Sedervedre

to the women who have honoured me in sharing the raw intensity of their birth space, who have stretched me to know more of my capacity, thank you for the lovely oxytocin.

notes

page 5: Archie Roach is an Indigenous Australian singer, songwriter and guitarist. I thank him for giving permission to use this quote.

page 21: The proportion of women giving birth by caesarean section continues to increase from 31.6 per cent in 2010 to 34.9 per cent in 2017 and 37 per cent in 2019. Report of the 2018–2021 Consultative Council on Obstetric and Paediatric Mortality and Morbidity (CCOPMM) https://www.bettersafercare.vic.gov.au/sites/default/files/2019-12/CCOPMM%20REPORT%20-%20FINAL_181219.pdf

page 47: Hospitals – from a submission to the Australian parliamentary inquiry into perinatal services 11/07/2017, written in conjunction with midwives Marie-Louise Lapeyre, Elizabeth Murphy and Samantha Ward.

page 53: *Policy* '...inside their lonely castles, broken hearts will dwell' is a line from the rock band Australian Crawl's song 'Hoochie Gucci Fiorucchi Mama'.

page 87: *Message tree*, crossing the branches of trees that continue to grow is a culturally significant practice of Indigenous cultures across Australia. The tree limbs are markers pointing in specific directions to important locations such as sources of water, food and sacred sites that connect the people to their traditional lands and culture.

page 127: *Birthing tree*, generations of Indigenous women birthed their babies within the burnt-out centres of ancestral birthing trees, planting their placentas in the ground around the trees, adding their blood and stories to these sacred, ancestral places.

photography

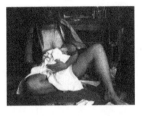

page 31
Author with Aidan
Photographer Dr Terri Labberton

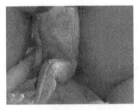 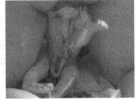 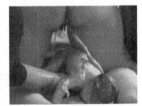

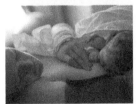

pages 62-65
Phoebe Barton with baby August
Photographer Jessie Boylan
www.jessieboylan.com

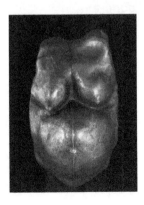

page 68
From a belly cast of my pregnancy with
Aidan, re-formed into this extraordinary
bronze modelled by Zoe Amor and cast
at the Garage Art Foundry.
Photographer Denise Martin
www.denisejmartin.net
www.zoeamor.com

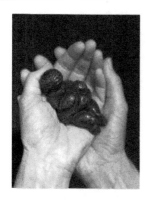

page 69
Doni for strength in birthing, bronze.
Gifted to me by Zoe Amor & Craig
MacDonald, on the birth of their daughter
Asha. Based on the so-called Venus of
Willendorf fertility figure made c. 28,000 –
25,000 BCE housed in the Naturhistorisches
Museum, Vienna, Austria.
Photographer Denise Martin

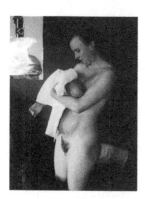

page 74
Katie Varallo, daughter Lily,
mother and grandmother
Photographer Lauren Starr
www.laurenstarr.com.au

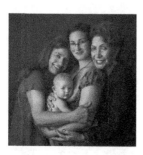

page 95
Author with Aidan,
wise woman watching over
Photographer Dr Terri Labberton

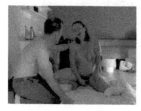 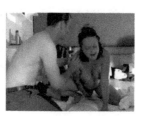 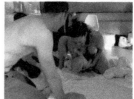

page 105-107
Lil Pearce, baby Esther and Will. Video stills by Milly Dubrowski

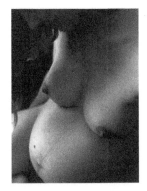

page 123
Author, pregnant with Jarah
Photographer Jacinta Barrow

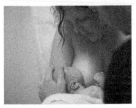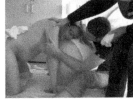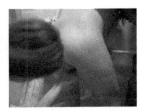

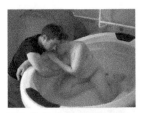

page 134-137
Amanda Bourdon, baby Finley and Heath
Photographer Breanna Gravener – The Birth
Story Photographer

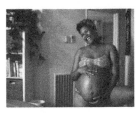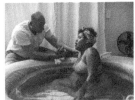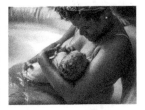

pages 152-154
Rusila Sevudredre, baby Solomon and Josh
Photographer Breanna Gravener

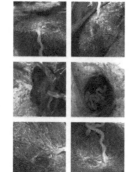

pages 174-175
Placenta images.
Photographer
Dr Veronica Moule

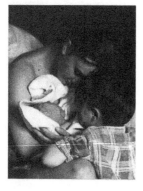

page 182
Author Aidan and Jarah.
Photographer Dr Terri Labberton

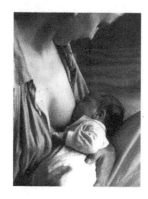

page 189
Author with Jarah
Photographer Jacinta Barrow